Second Edition

Manual of

Prescription Writing

with Case Scenarios

As per the latest NMC Guidelines | Competency Based Medical Education (CBME) Curriculum for the Indian Medical Graduate

Second Edition

Manual of Prescription Writing

with Case Scenarios

As per the latest NMC Guidelines | Competency Based Medical Education (CBME) Curriculum for the Indian Medical Graduate

Saroj Kothari
MBBS, MD (Pharmacology)
Professor and Head
Department of Pharmacology
Gajra Raja Medical College, Lashkar, Gwalior, MP
e-mail: saroj.kothari@rediffmail.com

Ashok Kumar Jain
MBBS
Senior Demonstrator
Department of Pharmacology
Gajra Raja Medical College, Lashkar, Gwalior, MP
e-mail: drashok77@gmail.com

CBSPD

CBS Publishers & Distributors Pvt Ltd

New Delhi • Bengaluru • Chennai • Kochi • Kolkata • Lucknow • Mumbai

Gujarat • Hyderabad • Jharkhand • Nagpur • Patna • Pune • Uttarakhand

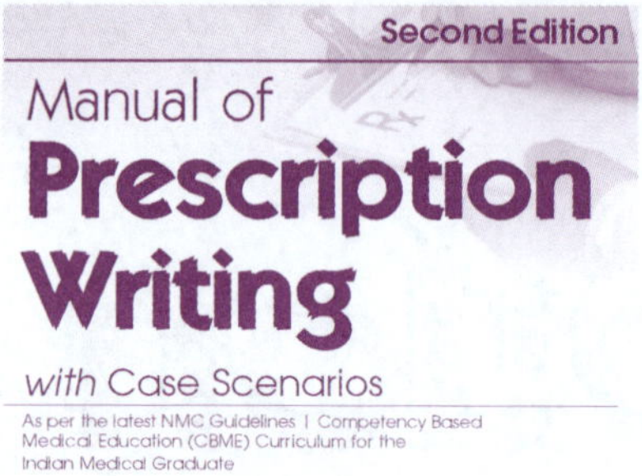

Disclaimer

Science and technology are constantly changing fields. New research and experience broaden the scope of information and knowledge. The authors have tried their best in giving information available to them while preparing the material for this book. Although all efforts have been made to ensure optimum accuracy of the material, yet it is quite possible some errors might have been left uncorrected. The publisher, the printer and the authors will not be held responsible for any inadvertent errors, omissions or inaccuracies.

ISBN:978-93-5466-601-8

Second Edition: 2024

Reprint: 2026

First Edition: 2021

Published by **Satish Kumar Jain**and produced by **Varun Jain**for

CBS Publishers & Distributors Pvt Ltd

4819/XI Prahlad Street, 24 Ansari Road, Daryaganj, New Delhi 110 002, India
Ph: 011-23289259, 23266838 Website: www.cbspd.com
e-mail: delhi@cbspd.com

Corporate Office: 204 FIE, Industrial Area, Patparganj, Delhi 110 092
Ph: 011-4934 4934 Fax: 011-4934 4935 e-mail: publishing@cbspd.com; publicity@cbspd.com

Branches

- **Bengaluru:**Seema House 2975, 17th Cross, KR Road, Banasankari 2nd Stage, Bengaluru 560 070, Karnataka, India
  Ph: +91-80-26771678/79 Fax: +91-80-26771680 e-mail: bangalore@cbspd.com
- **Chennai:**18/8B, Subbarayan Street, Shenoy Nagar, Chennai 600 030, Tamil Nadu, India
  Ph: +91-44-42032115, 45022115 e-mail: chennai@cbspd.com
- **Kochi:**42/1325, 1326, Power House Road, Opposite KSEB, 682 018, Kochi, Kerala, India
  Ph: +91-484-4059061-65 e-mail: kochi@cbspd.com
- **Kolkata:**147, Hind Ceramics Compound, 1st Floor, Nilgunj Road, Belghoria, Kolkata 700 056, West Bengal, India
  Ph: +91-33-25633055-56 e-mail: kolkata@cbspd.com
- **Lucknow:**Basement, Khushnuma Complex, 7-Meerabai Marg (behind Jawahar Bhawan), Lucknow 226 001, UP, India
  Ph: +91-522-4000032 e-mail: tiwari.lucknow@cbspd.com
- **Mumbai:**PWD Shed. Gala No. 25/26, Ramchandra Bhatt Marg, Next to JJ Hospital Gate No. 2
  Opposite Union Bank of India, Noorbaug, Mumbai 400 009, Maharashtra, India
  Ph: +91-22-66661880/89 e-mail: mumbai@cbspd.com

Representatives

• **Gujarat** • **Hyderabad** • **Jharkhand** • **Nagpur** • **Patna** • **Pune** • **Uttarakhand**

For trade terms please contact customercare@cbspd.com

For general enquiries please contact info@cbspd.com

Printed at Mudrak, Noida, UP, India

Preface to the Second Edition

With the implementation of CBME based curriculum in 2019 a need was felt to address the competency of prescribing. Efforts were made to clear doubts amongst second-phase MBBS students on how to write a correct prescription in our first edition of this book. It gives us immense pleasure to bring the second edition of this book for learners. This edition is revised and updated to incorporate current evidence-based drugs in prescriptions based on the standard treatment guidelines issued by WHO and other recognized professional scientific bodies. This will help to meet the expectations of the students. With our past experience and feedback from undergraduate and postgraduate students, some case scenarios of common ailments are included namely allergic conjunctivitis, anaemia in pregnancy, aphthous ulcer, COVID-19, dengue, dysmenorrhoea, GERD, generalized anxiety disorder, morning sickness, polycystic ovarian disease and urticaria. A checklist table is included for the critical appraisal of prescriptions. An alphabetical list of diseases covered for prescription writing is added as an appendix so that learners can quickly go through the case scenario and prescription. We would like to thank all our undergraduate and postgraduate students for their feedback. They provided great motivation to write the second edition of the book. We request the readers to give suggestions to improve the content given in this book to be incorporated in future.

We wish to express our gratitude to Mr YN Arjuna Senior Vice President—Publishing, Editorial and Publicity of CBS Publishers & Distributors Pvt. Ltd. for his continuous support, innovative ideas, and extraordinary cooperation to publish this work.

Saroj Kothari
Ashok Kumar Jain

Preface to the First Edition

"Your patients deserve the best and safest treatment and you deserve to have essential skills to deliver that care."

At the end of the second phase, it is found that most medical students are not confident of how to prescribe a drug to the patient or what information they need to provide. This is because earlier pharmacology training has focused more on theory than on practice. This method of teaching although helped in acquiring knowledge of pharmacology but failed to impart practical prescribing skills. Now National Medical Commission has introduced Competency Based Undergraduate Curriculum in 2019 therefore a need is felt to write this manual to impart competency of prescription writing in medical undergraduate second phase students. The knowledge students gain from textbook is difficult to retain and even more difficult is to recall this information when the clinical setting is encountered. Revised undergraduate medical education regulations (GMR, 2017) have focused on problem-based learning approach hence carefully constructed clinical case scenarios are given to teach prescription writing in this manual to fill the gap between basic science and clinical exposure. With the availability of so many drugs, at times many drug options are found suitable for a particular disease and the physicians choose the drug according to their experience. The general perception in students is that they will learn prescribing skills after completing the fourth phase of MBBS but research shows that there is a gain in experience, but prescribing skills do not improve much after graduation. It is well recognized that drug errors are a major cause of patient's morbidity and mortality, so good training is needed before poor habits get a chance to develop. To impart prescribing skill in students this manual is written with the following learning objectives:

1. Students should be able to understand the general principles of prescribing and able to write a complete and legible prescription for a given condition.
2. Students should be aware of some common errors of prescribing and able to correct them appropriately.
3. Students should be able to communicate with patients on prescriptions
4. Students should be able to perform a critical appraisal of a given prescription/ should know about prescription audit.
5. Students should be able to understand the legal and ethical aspects of prescribing.

This book covers the latest drugs to be prescribed for various diseases. It reflects credible information also on other suitable alternative options.

Medicine is an ever-changing science. With the day-to-day advancement in research and clinical experience, we need to update options of drug therapy. The authors and the publisher of this work have put in their best efforts to provide information that is complete and updated in accord with the standards accepted at the time of publication. Despite all efforts, there is the possibility of certain human errors or changes in medical sciences may have been overlooked. Therefore, neither the authors nor the publisher warrants that the information contained herein is in every respect accurate or complete, and they disclaim all responsibility for any errors or omissions or for the results obtained from the use of the information contained in this work. We wish the readers to confirm the information with other sources and refer to the manufacturer's recommendations for all dosages, especially for the new drugs. This book will serve as a resource for medical students/professionals, dental students, nurses, pharmacists and physiotherapists.

We acknowledge the feedback provided by our undergraduate, postgraduate students, pharmacology and medicine faculty members for the presentation of this manual. We are pretty sure that students will find this manual a tool to achieve the competency of safe prescribing. The authors would be grateful for any comments or constructive criticism to ensure that this manual continues to evolve and remains adapted to the reality of the field.

Saroj Kothari
Ashok Kumar Jain

Acknowledgements

With deep gratitude and respect we remember Almighty God for giving us the ability to understand, remember and write a book to impart prescribing skills in medical students.

We are thankful to our parents for their constant encouragement, love and care.

We are grateful to our teachers.

We are indebted to Prof (Dr) SP Dhaneria Sir, Academic Dean, Professor and Head, Department of Pharmacology, All India Institute of Medical Sciences, Raipur (CG), who consented to review the book and thankful to him for his valuable suggestions, support and encouragement.

We wish to express our thanks to our families for their support and encouragement.

We sincerely thank our departmental postgraduate students: Dr Ajay Gupta, Dr Vineet Chaturvedi, Dr Vaibhav Kalgaonkar, Dr Sanjay Kumar, Dr Seema Gogoi and Dr Jyoti Gadhvi for their feedback in preparing different chapters.

We wish to express our gratitude to Mr YN Arjuna Senior Vice President—Publishing, Editorial and Publicity of CBS Publishers & Distributors Pvt. Ltd. for accepting our proposal, continuous support, innovative ideas, extraordinary cooperation for publishing this book.

Saroj Kothari
Ashok Kumar Jain

Contents

Abbreviations

AST	After Sensitivity Test
bpm	Beats Per Minute
BP	Blood Pressure
Cap	Capsule
cm	Centimeter
e.g.	Example gratia, for example
etc.	Et cetera
g	Gram
Hb	Haemoglobin
Hg	Mercury
hr	Hour
hrly	Hourly
Inj	Injection
IM	Intramuscular
IV	Intravenous
kg	Kilogram
m	Month
max	Maximum
mm	Millimeter
mcg	Microgram
MDI	Metered Dose Inhaler
mg	Milligram
mL	Millilitre
min	Minutes
ng	Nanogram
pot	Potassium
sec	Seconds
SC	Subcutaneous
Sod	Sodium
Stat	Immediately
Tab	Tablet
wk	Week
wt	Weight
yr	Year

Chapter 1

General Considerations in Prescription Writing

Background

Once a patient is diagnosed with a disease and the practitioner opts for drug therapy, he has to select drugs from the available therapeutic options. This requires the writing of a prescription. A written prescription is an instruction or prescriber's order to a pharmacist to prepare and dispense a specific medicine for a particular patient. Prescriptions in the olden days were compounded and pharmacist used to prepare dosage forms. In modern times prescription drugs are precompounded and pharmaceutical companies supply different dosage forms of the drugs as per need. Presently prescription is an instruction from a prescriber to the patient and the dispenser.

The art of prescription writing is ancient. Originally its process was a little complex and written in the Latin language, subsequently replaced by English. The contemporary practice of prescribing is more systematic and simple. Every country has its own regulations of prescription; in fact there are no universal standards for this. Prescription is a legal document and is prima facie evidence in the court of law for which the prescriber is responsible. More often it is found that incomplete and incorrect prescriptions are handed over to the patients and also overlooked by pharmacists. This trend is putting patient safety at risk.

Prescription is an important intervention by the physician and it is the ethical and legal duty of the practitioner to write clearly and legibly. It should indicate precisely the drugs, dosage, route, timings and total quantity to be supplied.

Elements of Prescription

A prescription should be written in a systematic order. The correct prescription should contain the following elements:

1. *Doctor's particulars:* Name, professional degrees, address, telephone number and E-mail address of prescriber should be written or printed on top of the prescription paper. This will help the patient or pharmacist to contact the physician for any query or clarification. In government setup name of the hospital is printed on top of the prescription and the prescriber does his signature at the bottom. The size of the prescription paper should not be very small. The ideal minimum size is 14 × 21 cm (A5 size).

2. *Date:*Prescriptions should be dated at the time they are written. The date is important in creating the medication record of the patient and to check his compliance behaviour. The date is also important to pharmacist for dispensing of drugs prescribed under the Narcotic Drugs and Psychotropic Substances (NDPS) Act. To mention time along with date may be especially important while writing prescriptions for certain ailments, e.g. in case of poisoning or serious accidents/ illnesses.
3. *Patient's particulars:*Name, age, sex, weight and address of the patient should be written after prescriber's particulars. Patient's age, especially in paediatric and geriatric populations is required for proper drug and dose assurance. This step also helps to avoid age-inappropriate prescriptions. Patient's particulars are required so that the correct medication goes to the proper patient and also for identification and record-keeping purposes. Address of the patient is required so that he/she can be contacted if the need arises.
4. *Superscription:*It is a prescription symbol "R_X" written on the top left side of the body of prescription. This has been accepted all over the world as an invocational sign to the Jupiter who is considered as God of healing. The sign of Jupiter is employed as a request for healing. It represents the specific Latin verb "recipe" which means "take thou" or for you in the name of God.
5. *Inscription:*This is the most important part of the prescription. In this part, prescriber writes names of selected drugs in an order. The drug name should be written in capital letters. It is preferable to write generic names of drugs unless there are bioavailability issues. It is also important to mention medication strength, quantity to be taken and the duration. Computer typed prescriptions avoid errors due to bad handwriting.
6. *Subscription:*In this part of the prescription prescriber used to provide direction to the pharmacist regarding dispensing of preparation. Examples of prescription directions to the pharmacist are "make a mixture," "mix and place into 30 capsules". This part is no more applicable these days. Today, the majority of the prescriptions are written for medications already prepared as ready dosage forms by drug manufacturing industries.
7. *Transcription:*In this part, instructions to the patient are given like, to swallow or chew, shake well before use, to be taken with meals or on empty stomach, etc. This part comes just below the inscription. Renewal or refill instructions are written on the left side at the bottom. It is particularly important in the treatment of chronic diseases when the treatment is to be continued for a longer period. If refills are not allowed it should be clearly documented in prescription especially when drugs causing dependence are prescribed. In modern practice inscription, subscription and transcription are combined together.
8. *Signature:* The prescription ends with the signature of the doctor, date with his registration number and name of State Council or National Medical Commission under which he or she is registered. This will validate and authenticate the prescription. No blank space should be left between the body of the prescription and signature.

PRESCRIPTION FORMAT

R_x

Name of Dr. ----

Professional degree ----

Registration no. ------

Address------

Tel. no. ------

Date: -----

Email: -------@-----.com

Patient's name: -----------

Age & Sex: ------------

Weight : ------------

Address : -----------

Diagnosis: -----

R_x

Tab -----------

Refills ---

Signature

(Stamp)

MODEL PRESCRIPTION

A 30-year-old patient Mr. X weighing 45 kg was diagnosed as a case of generalized tonic clonic seizures. Write a prescription for this patient.

Dr XY Jain
MBBS, MD (Neurology)
Registration no. MPMC 223344
Family Wellness Clinic, Fort View, Gwalior, M.P.
Tel. no. 111222 Email: ---------@-------.com

Date: 10.01.2021

Patient's name: Mr X
Age & Sex: 30 years, Male
Weight: 45 kg
Address: 24, Modern Colony, Gwalior

Diagnosis: Generalized Tonic Clonic Seizures

R_x
Tab PHENYTOIN SODIUM 100 mg orally 12 hrly for 7 days
Review after 7 days
Avoid driving vehicles and operating machinery

Refills: None

XY Jain
Stamp

IMPORTANT POINTS FOR CORRECT AND SAFE PRESCRIBING

The prescription should be free of errors. Prescribing is a competency requiring knowledge of pharmacokinetics, pharmacodynamics and adverse drug reactions. The prescriber should also have a good memory and understanding of dosing and the ability to adapt the situation to an individual's circumstances. This all comes with experience. To prevent mistakes while prescribing the following points should be considered:

1. ***Accuracy and correctness:***The prescription is a legal record; hence it needs to be a correct and clear document written in English providing factual evidence of what occurred, as well as recordings of the accountable parties. These parties include

the prescriber and also the professional who administered the drug (pharmacist/ nurse). Side effects, adverse reactions, toxicity, drug interactions, and contraindications should be kept in mind while writing a prescription. It is, therefore, the doctor must take utmost precaution to make all prescriptions very clear and informative, as any mistake could be directly attributed to the prescriber however good the intention may be.

2. ***Name of drug:*** The international non-proprietary name or generic name of the drug should always be used. The trade name can be added if there is a specific reason to prescribe a special brand, e.g. drug with a specialized release system or a drug with a narrow therapeutic index. If it is handwritten prescription the name of the drug should be in capital letters so that the chances of errors due to bad handwriting are avoided however typed or computer generated prescriptions are better. Always write the correct spelling of the drug's name. Do not use abbreviations for drug names as these can be misinterpreted. For example, write Hyoscine methyl bromide, not HMN, Isosorbide dinitrate not IDN.
3. ***Approach medication names with caution:*** Names of drugs that look alike when spelt out and sound alike when spoken may contribute to dispensing errors, e.g.
   a. *Normace:* Norpace (Normace is Enalapril which is an antihypertensive drug while Norpace is Disopyramide which is an antiarrhythmic drug)
   b. *Neocare:* Neocalm (Neocare is Levodopa + Carbidopa used in Parkinsonism while Neocalm is Trifluoperazine used in Schizophrenia).
   c. *Isodril:* Isoprine (Isodril is Isosorbide dinitrate used in angina pectoris while Isoprine is Isoprenaline used in bradycardia).
4. ***Pharmaceutical dosage form of the drug:*** The pharmaceutical dosage form should be clearly stated, e.g. 'tablet', 'oral solution', 'eye ointment', 'vaginal pessary', etc. Each type of dosage form has unique pharmaceutical characteristics and designed for optimal drug action. When oral and injectable drugs are equally effective parenteral administration is only justified in case of emergency or when the patient is unable to take orally.
5. ***Dosage unit:*** The strength of the drug should be stated in standard units using abbreviations that are consistent with the System International (SI). Avoid common household measurements such as "teaspoons" or "tablespoons" as these are variable and cannot be reliable. 'Microgram' should not be abbreviated to µg, e.g. Clonidine 100 microgram or mcg but not µg. Also, 'units' should not be abbreviated, e.g. Injection Penicillin 4 Million Units, not MU to avoid confusion because U may be interpreted as 0 or 4.
6. ***Use of decimal points:*** Many errors in drug strength have occurred with unnecessary decimal points, e.g. write 100 mg, not 0.1 g, use leading zero before decimal point like write 0.4 mg and not .4 mg and avoid terminal zero after decimal point, e.g. write 8 mg, not 8.0 mg because it can resemble 80. When the strength of the drug is more than 1 g write the unit gram and for strength of the drug less than 1 g write the unit milligrams.
7. ***Dose frequency:*** The use of abbreviations in medication's frequency of administration is also a common source for medical errors. OD, BD, TDS and SOS though are

acceptable Latin abbreviations may work if all your patients are Latin scholars. Usually, these abbreviations confuse most of the patients. For example, it is better to write 12 hourly for BD. The drug with less frequent dosing should be preferred for better patient compliance. Dose frequency should be clear and explicit. The minimum dose interval should be stated together with the maximum daily dose for preparations given on 'as required' basis, where relevant. It is good practice to qualify such prescriptions with the purpose of the medication (for example '6 hourly as required for pain', 'at night as required for sleep'). Always specify times (6 a.m., 2 p.m., 10 p.m.) rather than simply frequency (three times a day) and especially relationship to meals for orally consumed medication.

8. ***Duration of therapy:*** Specify the therapeutic duration correctly. The number of prescribed pills should be matched to the expected duration of treatment and necessary reassessment visits. Write review dates for all antibiotic prescriptions.
9. ***Directions for patients:*** Write directions in easy English or in a language that the patient understands better. Avoid writing misleading or inappropriate directions such as 'take as directed' or 'take as before'. Provide clear and specific directions to reinforce treatment plans. The directions should be both drug-specific and patient-specific. Add additional instructions which guide patients to avoid medication adverse effects, e.g. take it with meals (Indomethacin), take the first dose before going to bed (Prazosin) and take while going to bed, e.g. Lorazepam.
10. ***Indication:*** It is mostly encouraged to write the indication of prescription. It helps the pharmacist to dispense appropriate medications and the patient to understand the drug's purpose.
11. ***Avoid polypharmacy:*** Limit each prescription to a minimum number of medications, since multiple drugs and instructions may overlap and confuse the pharmacist and the patient. It is likely that patients with multiple illnesses require multiple drugs even then attention should be paid to restrict polypharmacy.
12. ***Communication with patients:*** For proper use of prescribed medicines and better compliance communicate effectively with patients.
13. ***Refills and repeat prescription:*** It is necessary to ensure regular review of the patient for any adverse effects/ side-effects, ongoing need for this medication and if there is a need to change doses over time. The minimum duration between refills and number of refills should be clearly mentioned. Mention in prescription "do not refill" in case of drugs causing dependence.
14. ***Age of the patient:*** Do not forget to write the patient's age in order to check the correct dose. With the change in age there is a change in weight and body surface area, further in old age there is decline of renal and hepatic functions; all these age-related factors need to be considered for dose adjustment. Selection of drug is also age related, e.g. tetracycline is avoided in a child less than 8 years of age and lithium is avoided in the elderly. The patient's age orients pharmacists/chemists during their checks of appropriate drug and dose.
15. ***Record keeping:*** Always write prescriptions with ink which is indelible or cannot be cleaned or washed out. Any alterations should only be made in exceptional circumstances by rewriting and must be countersigned by the concerned doctor.

Blank prescription papers should be kept in a safe place to avoid misuse or prescription fraud. Never pre-sign a blank prescription. Regularly encircle your name when using preprinted prescription having names of more than one physician so the pharmacist will know whom to contact for corrections or clarifications. Always keep a copy of the prescription.

16. ***Documentation of drug allergy:*** This is important to avoid medication error or fatal consequences.

Chapter

2

Case Scenarios and Prescription Writing

INTRODUCTION

The medical world is expanding at a very fast pace. New drugs are continuously being developed and introduced in clinical practice to replace obsolete ones. A busy practitioner or a new degree holder in the medical profession should keep him abreast of these developments and reorient to the changing circumstances. Drug resistance is usually being encountered and is the main explanation for treatment failure.

In this small work, an attempt has been made to prescribe the most effective drugs for a specific disease. In the case of intolerance or allergic reaction or drug resistance, alternative regimens are also mentioned. However, the choice of drugs for a particular patient in a particular situation depends upon the treating physician.

Case scenarios of common ailments are given in alphabetical order for early clinical exposure of students and to initiate the thought process to make correct diagnosis and then to write drug/drugs of choice for that particular disease. The medications and the direction to the patients are written in a prescription format for a particular disease depicted in the case scenario. The *doctor's particulars, patient's particulars, date, signature and registration number of prescriber that are other essential elements of prescription are also mentioned for better understanding.* Along with main drug therapy, supplementary drugs are given for symptoms like fever, cough or vomiting, on as required basis in a particular case. Students should write complete prescription incorporating all the elements of prescription.

Drugs are prescribed preferably using generic names. Injectables are prescribed only when required and should be replaced by suitable oral drugs as soon as the patient is stable. As a general principle injectables are advised for a maximum period of 4 to 6 weeks and then therapy should be switched over to oral drugs if treatment is to be continued for a longer duration.

Reviews are also mentioned in those prescriptions where dose adjustment/ escalation/omission or addition of drugs are required during follow up care.

Refills are mentioned where the same treatment is to be continued after evaluation of the patient.

Prescriptions for Case Scenarios of Common Diseases

CASE SCENARIO 1

A 10-year-old boy named X presented to a neurologist after an episode of loss of consciousness that lasted for 10–20 seconds, with a blank stare, giddiness, eyelid fluttering and lip-smacking and dimness of vision. The patient reported that he regained from his loss of consciousness after a few seconds, however, the giddiness persisted. He experienced similar episodes quite sometimes in the past six months. His electroencephalogram (EEG) tracing showed a characteristic 3-Hz spike and dome pattern. Write a prescription for this patient incorporating all the elements.

Dr XY Jain
MBBS, MD (Paediatrics)
Registration no. MPMC 223344
25, Park Street, Gwalior MP
Tel. no. 111222 Email: -------@-----.com

Date: 10.01.2021

Patient's name: Mr X
Age & Sex: 10 years, Male
Weight: 25 kg
Address: 24, Modern Colony, Gwalior

Diagnosis: Absence Seizures

R_x
Cap Ethosuximide 250 mg orally 12 hrly for 7 days
Review after 7 days
Do not stop the drug without consulting doctor
Treatment is to be continued for 2–3 years after the last episode of seizure

XY Jain
Stamp

Alternative Agents

Tab Sodium Valproate 125 mg orally 12 hrly for 7 days OR
Tab Lamotrigine 25 mg ½ tab orally once daily

CASE SCENARIO 2

A 22-year-old female patient consulted a dermatologist with the complaints of multiple lesions over cheeks, chin, and forehead. She has had acne since she was a teenager and was treated with topical antibiotics and sunscreens without significant effect. On systemic examination, all the vital functions were normal. On local examination, multiple papulo-pustular lesions were present over cheeks, chin, and forehead. Under magnifying glass there were multiple blackhead and whitehead comedons. Write a prescription for this patient incorporating all the elements.

Dr XY Jain

MBBS, MD (General Medicine)

Registration no. MPMC 223344

25, Park Street, Gwalior MP

Tel. no. 111222 Email: -------@-----.com

Date: 00.00.0000

Patient's name: Ms X

Age & Sex: 22 years, Female

Address: .... Weight: ....

Diagnosis: Acne Vulgaris

R_X

Cap Doxycycline 100 mg orally 12 hrly for 2 weeks

Benzoyl Peroxide 2.5% Cream apply locally 12 hrly for 2 weeks

Take Doxycycline on empty stomach. Avoid dairy products, antacids and iron for two hr before and after Doxycycline

Avoid exposure to sunlight Review after 2 weeks

Refills: 2

XY Jain

Stamp

Alternative Agents

Cap Tetracycline 500 mg orally 12 hrly for 6 weeks OR

Tab Erythromycin 250 mg orally 6 hrly for 6 weeks OR

Tab Minocycline 50 mg orally 12 hrly for 6 weeks OR

Tab Trimethoprim/Sulfamethoxazole 160/800 mg orally 12 hrly for 6 weeks

CASE SCENARIO 3

A 58-year-old male was referred to a tertiary hospital with complaints of fever, chest pain, anorexia, weight loss, night sweats and productive cough with purulent sputum for 1 month. On examination, his temperature was 101.7°F and blood pressure was 150/80 mm Hg. Chest X-ray and CT scan showed necrosis and consolidation of the left lower lobe with pleural involvement. Bronchoalveolar lavage showed non-acid fast, gram-positive, branching, filamentous bacteria, identified as actinomycetes in culture on blood agar. Patient was admitted in medicine ward. Write a prescription for this patient incorporating all the elements.

Dr XY Jain
MBBS, MD (General Medicine)
Registration no. MPMC 223344
Family Wellness Clinic, Fort View, Gwalior, MP
Tel. no. 111222 Email: ---------@-------.com

Date: 00.00.0000

Patient's name: Mr X
Age & Sex: 58 years, Male
Address: .... Weight: ....

Diagnosis: Actinomycosis

R_X

Inj Penicillin G 3 Million Units IV 4 hrly for 6 weeks

Followed by

Tab Penicillin V 500 mg orally 6 hrly for 6 weeks to be taken 1 hr before or 2 hr after meals

Tab Paracetamol 500 mg orally 6–8 hrly as required for fever

Give first injection after sensitivity test (AST)

Review after 6 weeks

Refills: 2 for Tab Penicillin V

XY Jain
Stamp

Other First Line Agent in Place of Tab Penicillin V

Cap Amoxicillin 500 mg orally 6 hrly for 6 months

Alternative Agents to Penicillin G

Inj Ampicillin 3 g IV 6 hrly for 6 weeks

Followed by

Cap Amoxicillin 500 mg orally 8 hrly for 6 months OR
Cap Doxycycline 100 mg orally 12 hrly for 6 months

CASE SCENARIO 4

A 55-year-old man presents to a clinic with complaints of bloody, mucoid diarrhea for 4 days. On examination, his pulse is 90/minute and BP is 140/62 mm Hg. He has generalized abdominal tenderness. *Entamoeba histolytica* trophozoites were seen in stool samples. Write a prescription for this patient incorporating all the elements.

Dr XY Jain
MBBS, MD (General Medicine)
Registration no. MPMC 223344
Family Wellness Clinic, Fort View, Gwalior, MP
Tel. no. 111222 Email: ---------@-------.com

Date: 00.00.0000

Patient's name: Mr X
Age & Sex: 55 years, Male
Address: .... Weight: ....

Diagnosis: Acute Amoebic Dysentery

R_x
Tab Metronidazole 400 mg orally 8 hrly for 10 days

Followed by
Tab Diloxanide Furoate 500 mg orally 8 hrly for 10 days

XY Jain
Stamp

Alternative Agents to Metronidazole

Tab Tinidazole 2 g orally once daily for 3 days

Alternative Agents to Diloxanide Furoate

Tab Diiodohydroxyquin 650 mg orally 8 hrly for 21 days

CASE SCENARIO 5

A 28-year-old female presented to an ophthalmologist with complaints of redness, purulent discharge, irritation, burning, sticking of the eyelids upon waking and light sensitivity in both the eyes. The symptoms started 1 week ago; the right eye was affected first followed by left eye, 2 days later. On examination, bulbar conjunctiva was congested and mucopurulent discharge was present. Write a prescription for this patient incorporating all the elements.

Dr XY Jain
MBBS, MS (Ophthalmology)
Registration no. MPMC 223344
Family Wellness Clinic, Fort View, Gwalior, MP
Tel. no. 111222 Email: ---------@-------.com

Date: 00.00.0000

Patient's name: Ms X
Age & Sex: 28 years, Female
Address: .... Weight: ....

Diagnosis: Acute Bacterial Conjunctivitis

R_x
Moxifloxacin eye drops 0.5% 2 drops apply locally 6 hrly for 5 days

XY Jain
Stamp

Alternative Agents

Ofloxacin eye drops 0.3% 2 drops apply locally 4 hrly for 5 days OR
Ciprofloxacin eye drops 0.3% 2 drops apply locally 4 hrly for 5 days OR
Chloramphenicol eye drops 0.5% 2 drops apply locally 4 hrly for 5 days OR
Gentamicin eye drops 0.3% 2 drops apply locally 4 hrly for 5 days

CASE SCENARIO 6

A 26-year-old male presented with difficulty in breathing, wheezing, and cough. On examination, his pulse was 100/min, BP was 120/70 mm Hg and respiratory rate was 20/min. Chest auscultation revealed reduced breath sounds with prolonged expiration. On spirometry, FEV1 was 70% of predicted. Repeat spirometry after giving salbutamol recorded FEV1 as 90% of predicted. Write a prescription for this patient incorporating all the elements.

Dr XY Jain
MBBS, MD (General Medicine)
Registration no. MPMC 223344
Family Wellness Clinic, Fort View, Gwalior, MP
Tel. no. 111222 Email: ---------@-------.com

Date: 00.00.0000

Patient's name: Mr X
Age & Sex: 26 years, Male
Address: .... Weight: ....

Diagnosis: Acute Bronchial Asthma

R_X

Budesonide 100 mcg + Formoterol 6 mcg/puff. Inhale 2 puffs stat then repeat after 1 hr. (Max. 72 mcg of formoterol in 24 hrs)
Tab Bromhexine 8 mg orally 8 hrly
Review after 24 hr

XY Jain
Stamp

Alternative Agents

Terbutaline 250 mcg/puff by metered dose inhaler. Two puffs to be inhaled stat and then 1 puff 4 hrly if required.

CASE SCENARIO 7

A 34-year-old woman presents to her primary care physician with nasal congestion, sore throat, productive cough and fever for the last 4 days. Initially she was not short of breath, but now she becomes short of breath with exertion. She denies any hemoptysis. Auscultation of chest revealed diminished breath sounds. On physical examination, her temperature is 101.2°F with normal vital signs. On spirometry, FEV1 was 80% of predicted. Repeat spirometry after giving salbutamol recorded FEV1 as 85% of predicted. X-ray chest is normal. Write a prescription for this patient incorporating all the elements.

Dr XY Jain
MBBS, MD (General Medicine)
Registration no. MPMC 223344
Family Wellness Clinic, Fort View, Gwalior, MP
Tel. no. 111222 Email: ---------@-------.com

Date: 00.00.0000

Patient's name: Ms X
Age & Sex: 34 years, Female
Address: .... Weight: ....

Diagnosis: Acute Bronchitis

R_x

Cap Amoxycillin 500 mg orally 8 hrly for 5 days
Tab Bromhexine 8 mg orally 8 hrly for 5 days
Tab Paracetamol 500 mg orally 6–8 hrly as required for fever

XY Jain
Stamp

Alternative Agents

Tab Azithromycin 500 mg orally once daily for 3 days
Tab Cefuroxime 500 mg orally 12 hrly for 5 days OR
Tab Trimethoprim-Sulfamethoxazole (160/800 mg) orally 12 hrly for 5 days

CASE SCENARIO 8

A 46-year-old male presented with rapid onset of redness, pain and swelling in his right knee. Physical examination showed an obese man in acute distress with the following vital signs: Blood pressure 130/78 mm Hg, pulse 106 bpm, respirations 22/min, temperature 97.8°F. The patient's right knee was exquisitely tender and erythematous, warm to touch, and swollen with overlying skin tense, warm, and dusky red. The rest of the physical examination was normal. Blood test revealed raised uric acid. X-ray of the right knee showed soft tissue swelling around the joint but no erosion. Synovial fluid analysis showed needle and rod shaped strongly negative birefringent urate crystals both free in the fluid and engulfed by white blood cells. Write a prescription for this patient incorporating all the elements.

Dr XY Jain
MBBS, MD (General Medicine)
Registration no. MPMC 223344
Family Wellness Clinic, Fort View, Gwalior, MP
Tel. no. 111222 Email: ---------@-------.com

Date: 00.00.0000

Patient's name: Mr X
Age & Sex: 46 years, Male
Address: .... Weight: ....

Diagnosis: Acute Gout

R_X

Tab Ibuprofen 800 mg orally 8 hrly for 3 days then 400 mg 8 hrly for 4 days or until the pain is resolved

Review after 7 days

XY Jain
Stamp

Other First Line Agents

Tab Naproxen 500 mg orally 12 hrly for 3 days then 250 mg 12 hrly for 4 days or until the pain is resolved OR
Cap Indomethacin 50 mg orally 8 hrly for 3 days then 400 mg 8 hrly for 4 days or until the pain is resolved.

Alternative Agents: If NSAIDs Contraindicated

Tab Prednisolone: 40 mg orally once daily for 3 days
20 mg orally once daily for 2 days
10 mg orally once daily for 2 days

Note: When pain is not relieved by first line drugs
Tab Colchicine 1.2 mg followed by a dose of 0.6 mg 1 h later on the first day; thereafter dose for prophylaxis is 0.6 mg once or twice daily beginning 12 hr later until resolution. Max. 6 mg in 3–4 days.

CASE SCENARIO 9

A 60-year-old male was brought to emergency department with nausea, sweating and severe chest pain for 2 hr. The chest pain radiated to his left arm and jaw. His vital signs were blood pressure 124/80 mm Hg, pulse 110 bpm and regular, respirations 28/minute. ECG showed ST elevation in anterior leads. Patient was admitted in ICU. Write a prescription for this patient incorporating all the elements.

Dr XY Jain
MBBS, MD (General Medicine)
Registration no. MPMC 223344
25, Park Street, Gwalior MP
Tel. no. 111222 Email: -------@-----.com

Date: 00.00.0000

Patient's name: Mr X
Age & Sex: 60 years, Male
Address: .... Weight: ....

Diagnosis: Acute Myocardial Infarction

R_X
Complete bed rest for two days
Humidified O_2 inhalation
Tab Aspirin 150 mg orally once
Tab Clopidogrel 75 mg orally once
Tab Nitroglycerine 0.5 mg SL can repeat every 5 min for 3 doses
Tab Isosorbide Dinitrate 5 mg orally 4 hrly
Tab Metoprolol 50 mg orally 12 hrly
Inj Tenecteplase 30 mg IV bolus over 5 sec max dose 50 mg single dose
Inj Diazepam 10 mg IV once slowly
Inj Enoxaparin 40 mg SC once
Diet: Liquid diet on 1st day, salt restriction, semi-solid diet from 2nd day onwards.
Inj Pethidine 50 mg IV if pain not relieved by Nitroglycerine
To be reviewed after 24 hr

XY Jain
Stamp

CASE SCENARIO 10

A 45-year-old immunocompromised male injures his right thigh after falling to the ground. He sustained a piercing wound in thigh. He was given dressing for wound. Patient took analgesics for intense pain which subsides after taking drug but the pain returns off and on. The patient develops fever with chills after 5 days. He consults a physician next day. Physician notices that the lower right thigh is hot, swollen and tender. The right knee joint appears normal and has a full range of motion. The patient has a temperature 101.5°F. X-rays of the right femur indicates no obvious abnormalities of the bone. In blood test ESR and C-reactive protein are elevated. Blood cultures are positive for *Staphylococcus aureus*. Patient was admitted in orthopedic ward. Write a prescription for this patient incorporating all the elements.

Dr XY Jain
MBBS, MS (Orthopaedics)
Registration no. MPMC 223344
25, Park Street, Gwalior MP
Tel. no. 111222 Email: -------@-----.com

Date: 00.00.0000

Patient's name: Mr X
Age & Sex: 45 years, Male
Address: .... Weight: ....

Diagnosis: Acute Osteomyelitis

R_x
Inj Cefazoline 2 g IV 8 hrly for 7 days
Review after 7 days

XY Jain
Stamp

Alternative Agents

Inj Penicillin G 4 million units IV 6 hrly for 7 days OR
Inj Vancomycin 1 g IV 12 hrly for 7 days OR
Inj Clindamycin 900 mg IV 8 hrly for 7 days OR
Inj Oxacillin 2 g IV 6 hrly for 7 days

CASE SCENARIO 11

A 22-year-old female presented to her family physician with a 3-day history of rhinorrhea and a 2-day history of pain, fever and decreased hearing in right ear associated with fever. Her vital signs were normal except for an oral temperature of 101.5°F. On otoscopic examination of right ear the tympanic membrane was erythematous and bulging with decreased mobility. Write a prescription for this patient incorporating all the elements.

Dr XY Jain
MBBS, MS (ENT)
Registration no. MPMC 223344
25, Park Street, Gwalior MP
Tel. no. 111222 Email: -------@-----.com

Date: 00.00.0000

Patient's name: Ms X
Age & Sex: 22 years, Female
Address: .... Weight: ....

Diagnosis: Acute Otitis Media

R_X
Cap Amoxicillin 500 mg orally 8 hrly for 7 days
Tab Paracetamol 500 mg orally 6–8 hrly as required for fever

XY Jain
Stamp

Alternative Agents

Tab Azithromycin 500 mg orally once on day 1, followed by 250 mg once daily for 4 days OR

Tab Cephalexin 250 mg orally 8 hrly for 7 days OR

Tab Cefuroxime 250 mg orally 12 hrly for 7 days OR

Tab Trimethoprim/Sulfamethoxazole 160/800 mg orally 12 hrly for 5–7 days

CASE SCENARIO 12

A 42-year-old female presented with high fever, rigors, nausea, vomiting, dysuria, urinary frequency, urinary urgency and flank pain for 5 days. Physical examination revealed a temperature of 102° F, respiratory rate of 18 breaths per minute, heart rate of 108 beats per minute, blood pressure of 110/64 mm Hg. Her heart, lungs, and abdomen were normal, but there was mild costovertebral angle tenderness over the area of the left kidney. Urinalysis revealed large occult blood, proteinuria and 10 WBC/HPF (normal 0–3). A non-contrast computed tomography (CT) scan of the abdomen revealed severe left hydroureter and hydronephrosis without evidence of stones. Urine was sent for culture and sensitivity. Patient was admitted in medicine ward. Write a prescription for this patient incorporating all the elements.

Dr XY Jain
MBBS, MD (General Medicine)
Registration no. MPMC 223344
25, Park Street, Gwalior MP
Tel. no. 111222 Email: -------@-----.com

Date: 00.00.0000

Patient's name: Ms X
Age & Sex: 42 years, Female
Address: .... Weight: ....

Diagnosis: Acute Pyelonephritis

R_x
Inj Ceftriaxone 1 g IV once daily for 14 days
Tab Paracetemol 500 mg orally 6–8 hrly as required for fever

XY Jain
Stamp

Alternative Agents

Inj Piperacillin/Tazobactam 4.5 g IV 6 hrly for 10 days OR
Inj Cefoperazone/Sulbactam 3 g IV 12 hrly for 10 days OR
Inj Ciprofloxacin 400 mg IV 12 hrly for 14 days OR
Inj Gentamicin 240 mg IV once daily for 14 days OR
Inj Imipenem 500 mg IV 6 hrly for 10 days

CASE SCENARIO 13

A 30-year-old male presented with a history of alcohol intake over the last two years, with no periods of abstinence. The patient stated that he started drinking alcohol when he was 22-year-old along with his friends at college. Initially, he was taking alcohol two pegs, occasionally. Two year back his alcohol intake was increased due to his job pressure. He started having decreased sleep and appetite, irritability, tremors and poor concentration. He wanted to quit alcohol and was admitted in medicine ward. Write a prescription for this patient incorporating all the elements.

Dr XY Jain
MBBS, MD (General Medicine)
Registration no. MPMC 223344
25, Park Street, Gwalior MP
Tel. no. 111222 Email: -------@-----.com

Date: 00.00.0000

Patient's name: Mr X
Age & Sex: 30 years, Male
Address: .... Weight: ....

Diagnosis: Alcohol Addiction

R_x
Tab Disulfiram 500 mg orally once daily for 7 days followed by 250 mg orally once daily for 7 days
Tab Ondansetron 8 mg orally 8 hrly as required for vomiting
Review after 14 days

XY Jain
Stamp

Alternative Agents

Tab Naltrexone 50 mg orally once daily for 14 days
Tab Acamprosate 333 mg two tabs orally 8 hrly for 14 days

CASE SCENARIO 14

An 11-year-old male patient reports a four day history of irritation and itching first in the left eye followed by the right eye one day later. Eye examination revealed minimal redness in the eye with watering. The patient refused any foreign body sensation, flashes, deceased vision or diplopia. There was no history of trauma, surgery or contact lens use. The patient gave a family history of atopic disease. Write a prescription for this patient incorporating all the elements.

Dr XY Jain
MBBS, MS (Ophthalmology)
Registration no. MPMC 223344
25, Park Street, Gwalior MP
Tel. no. 111222 Email: ———@——.com

Date: 00.00.0000

Patient's name: Mr X
Age & Sex: 11 years, Male
Address: .... Weight: ....

Diagnosis: Allergic Conjunctivitis

R_x
Azelastine eye drops (0.05%) instill one drop per eye 12 hrly for five days
Review after 5 days

XY Jain
Stamp

Alternative Agents

Betamethasone eye drops (0.1%) instill one drop per eye 6 hrly

CASE SCENARIO 15

A 23-year-old female presented with sneezing, rhinorrhea, obstruction of the nasal passages, lacrimation and conjunctival, nasal and pharyngeal itching. Her symptoms started three days previously. On questioning, she told that her symptoms were worst in the late summer and in the early spring season. Examination revealed transverse nasal creases. The mucosa of the inferior turbinates was pale and oedematous with clear nasal secretion. Her eyes were both pink with conjunctival congestion. Write a prescription for this patient incorporating all the elements.

Dr XY Jain
MBBS, MD (General Medicine)
Registration no. MPMC 223344
25, Park Street, Gwalior MP
Tel. no. 111222 Email: -------@-----.com

Date: 00.00.0000

Patient's name: Ms X
Age & Sex: 23 years, Female
Address: .... Weight: ....

Diagnosis: Allergic Rhinitis

R_X
Beclomethasone nasal spray 50 mcg apply locally per nostril 12 hrly for 5 days
Tab Loratadine 10 mg orally once daily for 5 days

XY Jain
Stamp

Alternative Agents to Beclomethasone

Mometasone furoate nasal spray 200 mcg apply locally per nostril once daily for 5 days OR

Budesonide nasal spray 100 mcg apply locally per nostril 12 hrly for 5 days OR

Fluticasone propionate nasal spray 200 mcg apply locally per nostril once daily for 5 days.

Alternative Agents to Loratadine

Tab Desloratadine 5 mg orally once daily for 5 days OR

Tab Fexofenadine 120 mg orally once daily for 5 days OR

Tab Cetirizine 10 mg orally once daily for 5 days

CASE SCENARIO 16

A 72-year-old male is referred to a neurologist by his family physician as he has memory impairment for one year. He tells that his memory has worsened gradually over the last one year. The patient reports that he sometimes has difficulty finding the words he needs to express himself. He also has difficulty recalling the names of people, places or objects. Brain imaging with MRI is suggestive of neurodegenerative disease. Write a prescription for this patient incorporating all the elements.

Dr XY Jain
MBBS, MD (General Medicine)
Registration no. MPMC 223344
25, Park Street, Gwalior MP
Tel. no. 111222 Email: -------@-----.com

Date: 00.00.0000

Patient's name: Mr X
Age & Sex: 72 years, Male
Address: .... Weight: ....

Diagnosis: Alzheimer's Disease

R_X
Tab Donepezil 5 mg orally once daily for 4 weeks, then 10 mg daily for next 4 weeks
Review after 8 weeks

XY Jain
Stamp

Alternative Agents

Tab Galantamine 4 mg orally 12 hrly for 4 weeks, then 8 mg daily for next 4 weeks OR

Tab Memantine 5 mg orally once daily for 4 weeks, then 10 mg daily for next 4 weeks OR

Tab Rivastigmine 1.5 mg orally twice daily for 4 weeks, then 3 mg daily for next 4 weeks

CASE SCENARIO 17

A 15-year-old boy presents to his family physician with a sore throat and fever. He is diagnosed as a case of pharyngitis caused by group A β-hemolytic Streptococcus. He is given an IM injection of penicillin. Approximately 5 minutes later, he is found to be in respiratory distress and has audible wheezing. His heart rate is 110 per minute and his blood pressure is 70/30 mm Hg. Patient was admitted in medicine ward. Write a prescription for this patient incorporating all the elements.

Dr XY Jain
MBBS, MD (General Medicine)
Registration no. MPMC 223344
25, Park Street, Gwalior MP
Tel. no. 111222 Email: -------@-----.com

Date: 00.00.0000

Patient's name: Mr X
Age & Sex: 15 years, Male
Address: .... Weight: ....

Diagnosis: Anaphylactic Shock

R_X
Inj Adrenaline 1:1000 (1 mg/mL) 0.5 mL IM with repeated doses at 5–20 min intervals as needed for a severe reaction.
Inj Chlorpheniramine 10 mg IV stat
Inj Hydrocortisone 200 mg IV stat

XY Jain
Stamp

Alternative Route for Adrenaline

Inj Adrenaline 1:10000 (0.1 mg/mL) 0.5 mL IV slowly until response is achieved.

CASE SCENARIO 18

A 60-year-old male came to medical OPD with complaints of heaviness in chest that he experienced earlier in the day while climbing upstairs which was relieved after taking rest. He stated that such episodes occurred previously also on exertion or sometimes after taking large meals which were relieved after rest. His BP was 150/84 mm of Hg and pulse rate was 88/minute. ECG revealed mild ST depression. Patient was admitted in medicine ward. Write a prescription for this patient incorporating all the elements.

Dr XY Jain
MBBS, MD (General Medicine)
Registration no. MPMC 223344
25, Park Street, Gwalior MP
Tel. no. 111222 Email: -------@-----.com

Date: 00.00.0000

Patient's name: Mr X
Age & Sex: 60 years, Male
Address: .... Weight: ....

Diagnosis: Angina Pectoris

R_x

Tab Nitroglycerine 0.5 mg SL stat, if no relief then repeat same dose after 5 min till pain is relieved or for 3 doses
Tab Isosorbide Dinitrate 10 mg orally 8 hrly
Tab Aspirin 150 mg orally once daily
Tab Metoprolol 50 mg orally 12 hrly
Review after 24 hr

XY Jain
Stamp

Note: Further treatment of patient will depend on report of coronary angiography.

CASE SCENARIO 19

A 33-year-old woman complained of fatigue for 5 months. She is now 6 months pregnant. Her physical examination shows pale conjunctiva. The stool examination is negative for occult blood. Complete blood count shows Hb 9.0 mg/dL, haematocrit 23%, WBC 5400 cmm, platelet count 4.5 lacs/cmm, MCV 74 Fl (normal 84–95 Fl). Write a prescription for this patient incorporating all the elements.

Dr XY Jain
MBBS, MS (Obst. and Gynae)
Registration no. MPMC 223344
25, Park Street, Gwalior MP
Tel. no. 111222 Email: -------@-----.com

Date: 00.00.0000

Patient's name: Ms X
Age & Sex: 33 years, Female
Address: .... Weight: ....

Diagnosis: Anemia in pregnancy

R_x
Tab Ferrous Sulphate 300 mg once daily for 15 days
Tab Folic acid 5 mg orally once daily for 15 days
Review after 15 days
Oral iron makes the stool look black

XY Jain
Stamp

Alternative Agents

Tab Ferrous fumarate 180 mg orally once daily for 15 days OR
Tab Ferrous gluconate 500 mg orally once daily for 15 days

CASE SCENARIO 20

A 60-year-old man, living in rural area, presented with fever, malaise, headache, dyspnoea, cough, loss of appetite and myalgia for the last 15 days. The patient stated that he was treated with outpatient antibiotics a week ago but there was no improvement despite treatment. On physical examination, his temperature was 102.5°F, blood pressure was 150/80 mm Hg, pulse was 110/minute, and the respiratory rate 18/minute. Radiographic images showed mediastinal widening, bilateral pulmonary infiltrates and pleural effusion. Blood and sputum culture showed growth of *Bacillus anthracis* and the results were confirmed by polymerase chain reaction assay (PCR). Patient was admitted in medicine ward. Write a prescription for this patient incorporating all the elements.

Dr XY Jain
MBBS, MD (General Medicine)
Registration no. MPMC 223344
25, Park Street, Gwalior MP
Tel. no. 111222 Email: -------@-----.com

Date: 00.00.0000

Patient's name: Mr X
Age & Sex: 60 years, Male
Address: .... Weight: ....

Diagnosis: Anthrax

R_x

Inj Ciprofloxacin 400 mg IV 12 hrly till required and then switch to Tab Ciprofloxacin 500 mg orally 12 hrly until 60 days

Tab Paracetamol 500 mg orally 6–8 hrly as required for fever

XY Jain
Stamp

Alternative Agents

Inj Doxycycline 100 mg IV 12 hrly for 60 days (IV and oral combined) OR

Inj Penicillin G 12–20 Million Units AST IM once a day till required then switch to oral therapy when clinically stable with

Tab Ciprofloxacin 500 mg orally 12 hrly until 60 days

Note: For Cutaneous Anthrax treatment is given for 10 days.

CASE SCENARIO 21

A 10-year-old boy weighing 30 kg presented with colicky abdominal pain for 5 days. Abdominal USG showed multiple, long, linear, echogenic tubular structures in the ileal segment that were consistent with *A. lumbricoides* infestation. Stool testing showed a large number of *A. lumbricoides* eggs. Write a prescription for this patient incorporating all the elements.

Dr XY Jain
MBBS, MD (Paediatrics)
Registration no. MPMC 223344
25, Park Street, Gwalior MP
Tel. no. 111222 Email: -------@-----.com

Date: 00.00.0000

Patient's name: Mr X
Age & Sex: 10 years, Male
Weight: 30 kg
Address: .... Weight: ....

Diagnosis: Ascariasis

R_X
Tab Albendazole 400 mg orally single dose

XY Jain
Stamp

Alternative Agents

Tab Mebendazole 100 mg orally 12 hrly for 3 days OR
Tab Pyrantel Pamoate 250 mg orally single dose OR
Tab Ivermectin 6 mg orally single dose

CASE SCENARIO 22

A 46-year-old male presented with sudden onset of breathlessness after a 5-day history of productive cough, chest discomfort and fever. On examination, he was febrile and tachypnoeic, with oxygen saturation of 84% on high-flow oxygen. Respiratory system examination showed bronchial breath sounds in the right supraclavicular and interscapular areas. All other systems were within normal limits. X-ray chest showed a round infiltration in the upper part of the right lung. Direct microscopic examination of the sputum showed septate hyphae compatible with a filamentous fungus. A high-resolution CT scan of the chest showed a localized ground-glass appearance around a consolidation (halo sign) suggestive of invasive aspergillosis. Fine needle lung biopsy was performed and culture grew *Aspergillus* species. Write a prescription for this patient incorporating all the elements.

Dr XY Jain
MBBS, MD (General Medicine)
Registration no. MPMC 223344
25, Park Street, Gwalior MP
Tel. no. 111222 Email: -------@-----.com

Date: 00.00.0000

Patient's name: Mr X
Age & Sex: 46 years, Male
Address: .... Weight: ....

Diagnosis: Aspergillosis

R_X
Tab Voriconazole 200 mg orally 12 hrly for 6 weeks

XY Jain
Stamp

Alternative Agents

Tab Itraconazole 200 mg orally 12 hrly for 6 weeks OR
Tab Isavuconazole 200 mg orally once daily for 6 weeks OR
Tab Posaconazole 300 mg orally 12 hrly on day 1 and then 300 mg once daily for 6 weeks

CASE SCENARIO 23

A 35-year-old male patient complains of pain and a burning sensation in a localised area of the mucosa of the upper palate more so after eating spicy food for 3 days. There is no history of fever or drug intake. The patient gives a negative history of tobacco intake or smoking. On examination, there is a small lesion found on the mucosa of the upper palate and it does not bleed on touch. The histopathological examination does not reveal any malignancy. Write a prescription for this patient incorporating all the elements.

Dr XY Jain
MBBS, MD (General Medicine)
Registration no. MPMC 223344
25, Park Street, Gwalior MP
Tel. no. 111222 Email: -------@-----.com

Date: 00.00.0000

Patient's name: Mr X
Age & Sex: 35 years, Male
Address: .... Weight: ....

Diagnosis: Aphthous ulcer

Rx
Capsule B complex orally once daily for 5 days
Gel Choline salicylate for local application 6 hourly for 5 days before meals
Put 1–2 drops of gel on clean index finger and rub gently over affected area
Avoid eating oily and spicy food

XY Jain
Stamp

Alternative Agents

Lignocaine 2% viscous gel for local application before meals

CASE SCENARIO 24

A 35-year-old male presents with fever, headache, malaise, sore throat and cough. He was well until 3 days earlier, when he suffered from mild sore throat and productive cough with small amount of clear sputum. On examination, his temperature is 101°F, pulse 102 beats/min, BP 110/70 mm Hg, respiratory rate 18 beats/min. On auscultation, inspiratory crackles and bronchial breath sounds are present. The chest radiograph shows pneumonic consolidation on the right upper lung field. Anti-Mycoplasma IgM antibodies are present at a titer of 1:160 in serologic test and *Mycoplasma pneumoniae* is detected in respiratory tract secretions in polymerase chain reaction (PCR) test. Write a prescription for this patient incorporating all the elements.

Dr XY Jain
MBBS, MD (General Medicine)
Registration no. MPMC 223344
25, Park Street, Gwalior MP
Tel. no. 111222 Email: -------@-----.com

Date: 00.00.0000

Patient's name: Mr X
Age & Sex: 35 years, Male
Address: .... Weight: ....

Diagnosis: Atypical Pneumonia

R_x
Tab Azithromycin 500 mg orally as a single dose on day 1, followed by 250 mg orally once a day on days 2 to 5
Tab Bromhexine 8 mg orally 8 hrly as required for cough or for 7 days
Tab Paracetamol 500 mg 6–8 hrly as required for fever

XY Jain
Stamp

Alternative Agents

Tab Clarithromycin 500 mg orally 12 hrly for 14 days OR
Cap Doxycycline 100 mg orally 12 hrly for 14 days OR
Tab Levofloxacin 750 mg orally once daily for 14 days OR
Tab Moxifloxacin 400 mg orally once daily for 14 days

CASE SCENARIO 25

An 80-year-old man presented with a 1-year history of increased frequency of micturition, urgency, nocturia, poor stream, sensation of incomplete bladder emptying, straining to urinate, and post-void dribbling. Digital rectal examination revealed an enlarged, firm prostate without nodules or tenderness. The estimated total serum prostate specific antigen (PSA) level was 3.1 ng/mL. The prostatic volume measured by transrectal ultrasound was 55 mL. Write a prescription for this patient incorporating all the elements.

Dr XY Jain
MBBS, MS (General Surgery)
Registration no. MPMC 223344
25, Park Street, Gwalior MP
Tel. no. 111222 Email: -------@-----.com

Date: 00.00.0000

Patient's name: Mr X
Age & Sex: 80 years, Male
Address: .... Weight: ....

Diagnosis: Benign Prostatic Hyperplasia

R_X
Tab Silodosin 4 mg orally once daily for 1 month
Tab Dutasteride 0.5 mg orally once daily for 1 month
Review after 1 month

XY Jain
Stamp

Alternative Agents to Silodosin

Cap Tamsulosin 0.4 mg orally once daily for 1 month OR
Tab Alfuzosin 10 mg orally once daily for 1 month

Alternative Agents to Dutasteride

Tab Finasteride 5 mg orally once daily for 1 month

CASE SCENARIO 26

A 24-year-old male presented to a psychiatrist with a history of marked mood swings between depression and mania. The cycle had begun two year previously following a suicidal attempt. During his depressive periods, he was apathetic, retarded and extremely drowsy. He felt that he was worthless, had no motivation, and lacked energy. He felt more distressed in crowded places. When manic he had higher levels of self-confidence, got more sociable with strangers, was more talkative, behaved aggressively, showed a flight of ideas, elation, distractibility and constant restless movements. He had no hallucinations or delusions, and his cognitive state was unimpaired. The swing between the two moods was relatively fast and reliable, showing periodicity of about four to five weeks. His blood tests, including a complete blood count and thyroid function tests, were normal. Write a prescription for this patient incorporating all the elements.

Dr XY Jain
MBBS, MD (Psychiatry)
Registration no. MPMC 223344
25, Park Street, Gwalior MP
Tel. no. 111222 Email: -------@-----.com

Date: 00.00.0000

Patient's name: Mr X
Age & Sex: 24 years, Male
Address: .... Weight: ....

Diagnosis: Bipolar Disorder

R_x
Tab Lithium carbonate 300 mg orally 8 hrly for 15 days
Review after 15 days

XY Jain
Stamp

Alternative Agents

Tab Divalproex Sodium 500 mg orally 12 hrly for 30 days OR
Tab Carbamazepine 200 mg orally 12 hrly for 30 days OR
Tab Lamotrigine 50 mg orally once daily for 30 days

CASE SCENARIO 27

A 23-year-old male presented with complaints of high-grade intermittent fever with chills and rigors, malaise, fatigue, myalgias and loss of appetite of four weeks duration. There was an evening rise of temperature. He was investigated many times and treated with antimalarials and various antibiotics without any significant relief. On examination, he had a temperature of 101°F and pulse rate of 108 beats/minute. Haematology revealed haemoglobin of 11.4 gm%, total white blood cell count of 5200 cells/mm^3 and ESR 28 mm at one hr. Ultrasound of the abdomen showed mild splenomegaly. ELISA test for Brucella IgM antibodies was positive. Blood culture yielded growth of *Brucella melitensis* and was confirmed by polymerase chain reaction (PCR). Write a prescription for this patient incorporating all the elements.

Dr XY Jain
MBBS, MD (General Medicine)
Registration no. MPMC 223344
25, Park Street, Gwalior MP
Tel. no. 111222 Email: -------@-----.com

Date: 00.00.0000

Patient's name: Mr X
Age & Sex: 23 years, Male
Address: .... Weight: ....

Diagnosis: Brucellosis

R_x
Inj Streptomycin 1 g IM once daily for 21 days
Cap Doxycycline 100 mg orally 12 hrly for 6 weeks
Tab Paracetamol 500 mg orally 6–8 hrly as required for fever

XY Jain
Stamp

Alternative Agents to Streptomycin

Tab Rifampicin 600 mg orally once daily for 6 weeks OR
Inj Gentamicin 240 mg IM once daily for 14 days

CASE SCENARIO 28

A 35-year-old male presented with painful penile lesions that had progressed for approximately two weeks prior to presentation. The patient reported unprotected sex with multiple partners. The patient stated that the lesions began as small erythematous macules that slowly progressed to form ulcers. The man's vital signs were normal. The physical examination revealed three painful, soft ulcers on penis, with a necrotic base, surrounding erythema, and undermined edges associated with tender inguinal lymphadenopathy. Culture of a swab of the lesion was positive for *Haemophilus ducreyi*. Write a prescription for this patient incorporating all the elements.

Dr XY Jain
MBBS, MD (General Medicine)
Registration no. MPMC 223344
25, Park Street, Gwalior MP
Tel. no. 111222 Email: -------@-----.com

Date: 00.00.0000

Patient's name: Mr X
Age & Sex: 35 years, Male
Address: .... Weight: ....

Diagnosis: Chancroid

R_x
Tab Azithromycin 1 g orally as single dose

XY Jain
Stamp

Alternative Agents

Inj Ceftriaxone 250 mg IM single dose OR
Tab Ciprofloxacin 500 mg orally 12 hrly for 3 days OR
Tab Erythromycin 500 mg orally 6 hrly for 7 days

CASE SCENARIO 29

A 32-year-old woman presents to a hospital with a history of sudden onset of severe diarrhoea and vomiting for one day. She also complains of profound weakness. She has just returned from a trip to a remote village where she worked for two days in a camp. There she developed intestinal gurgling and vomiting followed by three loose bowel movements. Soon she was having profuse watery diarrhoea occurring frequently. The liquid stools are grey, turbid, and without faecal odour, blood, or pus. She looks very weak but has no fever. Blood pressure is 100/60 mm Hg. *V. cholerae* are identified in stool examination directly by darkfield microscopy on a wet mount of fresh stool. Write a prescription for this patient incorporating all the elements.

Dr XY Jain
MBBS, MD (General Medicine)
Registration no. MPMC 223344
25, Park Street, Gwalior MP
Tel. no. 111222 Email: -------@-----.com

Date: 00.00.0000

Patient's name: Ms X
Age & Sex: 32 years, Female
Address: .... Weight: ....

Diagnosis: Cholera

Rx
Cap Doxycycline 300 mg orally single dose
Tab Metoclopramide 10 mg orally 8 hrly as required

XY Jain
Stamp

Alternative Agents

Tab Azithromycin 1 g orally once daily for 3 days OR
Tab Ciprofloxacin 500 mg orally 12 hrly for 3 days

CASE SCENARIO 30

A 50-year-old man presented to the urology clinic complaining of urinary urgency, dysuria, frequency and urethral discharge. He also complained of suprapubic pain during voiding. He gave history of similar episodes frequently during the last one year which were relieved by brief courses of antibiotics prescribed by his family physician. On examination, his vital signs were normal. Per rectal examination showed a painful, enlarged, symmetrical smooth prostate. Cystoscopic examination revealed prostatic enlargement with congested prostatic mucosa suggestive of chronic prostatitis. Culture of urine obtained after prostatic massage was positive for *Proteus mirabilis*. Write a prescription for this patient incorporating all the elements.

Dr XY Jain
MBBS, MD (General Medicine)
Registration no. MPMC 223344
25, Park Street, Gwalior MP
Tel. no. 111222 Email: -------@-----.com

Date: 00.00.0000

Patient's name: Mr X
Age & Sex: 50 years, Male
Address: .... Weight: ....

Diagnosis: Chronic Bacterial Prostatitis

R_X
Tab Ciprofloxacin 500 mg orally 12 hrly for 28 days

XY Jain
Stamp

Alternative Agents

Tab Levofloxacin 500 mg orally once daily for 28 days OR
Cap Doxycyclin 100 mg orally 12 hrly for 28 days OR
Tab Azithromycin 500 mg orally once daily for 28 days OR
Tab Trimethoprim/Sulfamethoxazole (160/800 mg) orally 12 hrly for 28 days

CASE SCENARIO 31

A 60-year-old male presents with progressive shortness of breath on exertion for the past several days. His present problem began five days ago when he developed sore throat, rhinorrhea and myalgia. Later he developed a productive cough with mucopurulent sputum. He reports that he developed similar symptoms six months ago and he was diagnosed with acute bronchitis by his family physician and was treated. Patient had similar episodes frequently over the past six months. He had a 20 year history of smoking a pack of cigarettes a day however; he quit smoking shortly prior to the onset of symptoms. On examination, his blood pressure is 134/82 mmHg, heart rate is 96/minute, respiratory rate is 28/minute and temperature is 100.2°F. Examination of the chest reveals bilaterally diminished breath sounds with coarse crackles. On spirometry FEV1/FVC is less than normal. Write a prescription for this patient incorporating all the elements.

Dr XY Jain
MBBS, MD (General Medicine)
Registration no. MPMC 223344
25, Park Street, Gwalior MP
Tel. no. 111222 Email: -------@-----.com

Date: 00.00.0000

Patient's name: Mr X
Age & Sex: 60 years, Male
Address: .... Weight: ....

Diagnosis: Chronic Bronchitis

R_x
Tab Amoxicillin/Clavulanic acid 500/125 mg orally 8 hrly for 7 days
Tab Bromhexine 8 mg orally 8 hrly for 7 days
Tab Paracetamol 500 mg 6–8 hrly as required for fever

XY Jain
Stamp

Alternative Agents

Tab Cefuroxime 500 mg orally 12 hrly for 7 days OR
Tab Doxycyclin 100 mg orally 12 hrly for 7 days OR
Tab Trimethoprim Sulfamethoxazole (160/800 mg) orally 12 hrly for 7 days OR
Tab Azithromycin 500 mg orally on day 1 followed by 250 mg orally daily for 4 days OR
Tab Levofloxacin 500 mg orally once daily for 7 days OR
Tab Moxifloxacin 400 mg orally once daily for 7 days

CASE SCENARIO 32

A 62-year-old male presented with gouty arthritis for 7 year. He was taking colchicine and urate-lowering drug for the last 7 year but he was noncompliant with the therapy. On physical examination, he had massive and deforming tophi and active synovitis of bilateral small joints of the hands, wrists, elbows, knees and ankles. There were ulcerated lesions over the tophi in both ankles. Laboratory data revealed uric acid 8.3 mg/dL and C-reactive protein 7.8 mg/dL. X-ray of hands showed erosion. Write a prescription for this patient incorporating all the elements.

Dr XY Jain
MBBS, MD (General Medicine)
Registration no. MPMC 223344
25, Park Street, Gwalior MP
Tel. no. 111222 Email: -------@-----.com

Date: 00.00.0000

Patient's name: Mr X
Age & Sex: 62 years, Male
Address: .... Weight: ....

Diagnosis: Chronic Gout

R_x
Tab Allopurinol 100 mg orally once daily from 1st to 7th day then
200 mg orally once daily from 8th to 14th day
300 mg orally once daily from 15th to 21st day
Tab Paracetamol 500 mg orally 8 hrly as required for pain
Drink at least 10 glasses of water daily.

XY Jain
Stamp

Alternative Agents

Tab Febuxostat 40 mg orally once daily for 21 days

CASE SCENARIO 33

A 25-year-old healthy female, married two months back, attends gynaecology OPD. She does not want to become pregnant for 2 year. Her menstrual cycle is of 28 days and menstruation lasts for 4–5 days. Her clinical examination including blood pressure was normal. Write a prescription for this woman.

Dr XY Jain
MBBS, MS (Obstetrics & Gynaecology)
Registration no. MPMC 223344
25, Park Street, Gwalior MP
Tel. no. 111222 Email: -------@-----.com

Date: 00.00.0000

Patient's name: Ms X
Age & Sex: 25 years, Female
Address: .... Weight: ....

Diagnosis: Advice for Contraception

R_x
Tab Norgestrel + Ethinyl Oestradiol 300 mcg/30 mcg once daily from 5th day of menstrual period for 21 days.
Repeat same course after 7 days every month
Take one pill before going to bed daily uninterruptedly.
Report if more than two tablets are missed
Take colored iron tablets for 7 days after hormonal pills.
Refill every month for 23 months

XY Jain
Stamp

Alternative Agents

Tab Levonorgestrel 150 mcg + Tab Ethinyl Oestradiol 30 mcg orally once daily from 5th day of menstrual period for 21 days

CASE SCENARIO 34

A 57-year-old female patient, weighing 60 kg presented to the emergency department of hospital, with a history of fever and headache for the last two weeks and neck rigidity for the last 3 days. On examination, she had photophobia and a temperature of 102.5°F. A brain computed tomography scan was carried out but did not reveal any abnormal findings. Cerebrospinal fluid (CSF) examination under direct microscopy, following India ink preparation, detected multiple encapsulated yeast cells, typical of *C. neoformans*. CSF culture also showed growth of *Cryptococcus neoformans*. Write a prescription for this patient incorporating all the elements.

Dr XY Jain
MBBS, MD (General Medicine)
Registration no. MPMC 223344
25, Park Street, Gwalior MP
Tel. no. 111222 Email: -------@-----.com

Date: 00.00.0000

Patient's name: Ms X
Age & Sex: 57 years, Female
Weight: 60 kg
Address: ....

Diagnosis: Cryptococcal Meningitis

R_x

Inj Amphotericin B 50 mg in 500 mL of 5% dextrose, initially 10 mL IV slowly in 30 min to check sensitivity if tolerated then 3 mL/min once daily for 2 weeks
Cap Flucytocine 250 mg orally 6 hrly for 2 weeks
Tab Paracetamol 500 mg orally 6–8 hrly as required for fever.
Review after 2 weeks

XY Jain
Stamp

Note: Flucytocine is followed by:
Tab Fluconazole 400 mg orally once daily for 12 weeks
then Tab Fluconazole 200 mg orally once daily to complete one year therapy.

CASE SCENARIO 35

A 64-year-old male presents with complaints of left lower extremity pain that is worse on walking. The patient has no chest pain or shortness of breath. He states that a left total knee replacement was performed two weeks ago. Upon physical examination the patient's left calf is erythematous and swollen with dusky appearance and pitting oedema is present in the left lower extremity extending into the patient's thigh. Localized tenderness is also noted upon light palpation. The total knee replacement incision is healing and well approximated without any drainage. A Doppler ultrasonography of the left leg reveals left popliteal vein thrombosis extending into the superficial femoral vein. Write a prescription for this patient incorporating all the elements.

Dr XY Jain
MBBS, MS (General Surgery)
Registration no. MPMC 223344
25, Park Street, Gwalior MP
Tel. no. 111222 Email: -------@-----.com

Date: 00.00.0000

Patient's name: Mr X
Age & Sex: 64 years, Male
Address: .... Weight: ....

Diagnosis: Deep Vein Thrombosis

R_X
Inj Enoxaparin 60 mg SC 12 hrly for 5 days
Followed by
Tab Dabigatran 150 mg orally 12 hrly for 4 weeks
Tab Paracetamol 500 mg orally 6–8 hrly as required for pain
Review after 5 days

XY Jain
Stamp

Alternative Agents

Inj Dalteparin 200 International Units/kg SC once daily for 5 days OR
Inj Tinzaparin 175 International Units/kg SC once daily for 5 days

Followed by
Tab Dabigatran 150 mg orally 12 hrly for 4 weeks OR
Tab Edoxaban 60 mg orally once daily for 4 weeks

CASE SCENARIO 36

A 35-year-old female presents to a physician with complaints of fatigue. She states that she has daily crying spells, feels sad "all the time" and, not sleeping well and is overeating. She reports that her sleeping pattern has also been altered and it frequently takes her several hours to fall asleep. She reveals that she is constantly thinking and worrying. She denies suicidal behavior and ideations. Her physical examination is normal. Her blood tests, including a complete blood count and thyroid function tests, are normal. Write a prescription for this patient incorporating all the elements.

Dr XY Jain
MBBS, MD (Psychiatry)
Registration no. MPMC 223344
25, Park Street, Gwalior MP
Tel. no. 111222 Email: -------@-----.com

Date: 00.00.0000

Patient's name: Ms X
Age & Sex: 35 years, Female
Address: .... Weight: ....

Diagnosis: Depression

R_x
Tab Fluoxetine 20 mg orally 12 hrly for 15 days
Review after 15 days

XY Jain
Stamp

Alternative Agents

Tab Venlafaxine 200 mg orally once daily for 15 days OR
Tab Escitalopram 10 mg orally once daily for 15 days OR
Tab Sertraline 25 mg orally once daily for 15 days

CASE SCENARIO 37

A 56-year-old male patient weighing 85 kg came to the OPD with complaints of frequency of urination and easy fatigability. His fasting blood sugar was 124 mg/dL, postprandial blood glucose 188 mg/dL and HbA1C 7.2%. His blood pressure was 130/80. His father was diabetic. His fasting blood glucose 6 months back was normal. Write a prescription for this patient incorporating all the elements.

Dr XY Jain
MBBS, MD (General Medicine)
Registration no. MPMC 223344
25, Park Street, Gwalior MP
Tel. no. 111222 Email: -------@-----.com

Date: 00.00.0000

Patient's name: Mr X
Age & Sex: 56 years, Male
Weight: 85 kg
Address: ....

Diagnosis: Diabetes Mellitus Type II

R_x
Tab Metformin 500 mg orally 12 hrly with meals for 7 days
Reduce weight
Brisk walking for at least 30 min daily
Review after 7 days for dose titration as per blood glucose level

XY Jain
Stamp

CASE SCENARIO 38

A 45-year-old male complains of fever, pain in throat, cough and bodyache for 3 days. There is no history of chills and rigors, vomiting, pain in abdomen and joint pains. The patient gave a history of travel to Kerala. RT-PCR for the coronavirus is positive. Oxygen saturation using a pulse oximeter was recorded as 95%. HRCT, CRP, LDH, IL6, and D-dimer are normal. Write a prescription for this patient incorporating all the elements.

Dr XY Jain
MBBS, MD (General Medicine)
Registration no. MPMC 223344
25, Park Street, Gwalior MP
Tel. no. 111222 Email: -------@-----.com

Date: 00.00.0000

Patient's name: Mr X
Age & Sex: 45 years, Male
Address: .... Weight: ....

Diagnosis: COVID-19

R_x

Isolate yourself in self ventilated room
Tab Paracetamol 500 mg orally 6–8 hrly as required for fever
Tab Azithromycin 500 mg orally once daily for 3 days
Tab Vitamin C 500 mg orally once daily
Tab Zinc 20 mg orally once daily
Syp Dextromethorphan hydrobromide (15 mg/5 ml) 10 ml orally 8 hrly
Use triple layer mask
Take rest
Drink plenty of fluid orally
Frequent hand washing with soap and water or Clean hands with alcohol based sanitizer
Measure oxygen saturation 8 hrly

XY Jain
Stamp

CASE SCENARIO 39

A 29-year-old male with type I diabetes since the age of 13 year was brought to emergency department with a history of fever, cough, vomiting and drowsiness since 4 hr. On examination, his respiratory rate was 24/min and tongue was dry and coated. His temperature was 101°F. His blood sugar was 500 mg/dL, arterial pH was 6.7. Urine examination was positive for ketone bodies. Patient was admitted in medicine ICU. Write a prescription for this patient incorporating all the elements.

Dr XY Jain
MBBS, MD (General Medicine)
Registration no. MPMC 223344
25, Park Street, Gwalior MP
Tel. no. 111222 Email: -------@-----.com

Date: 00.00.0000

Patient's name: Mr X
Age & Sex: 29 years, Male
Address: .... Weight: ....

Diagnosis: Diabetic Ketoacidosis

R_X

Inj Regular Insulin 5 Units IV stat Followed by 5 Units IV infusion/hr for 6 hr

Followed by 2 Units/hr till the patient becomes fully conscious then switch to SC insulin

Normal saline 0.9% IV at the rate of 1 L/hr, followed by 5% Glucose in 0.45% saline after the blood sugar has reached 300 mg/dL

Inj Pot Chloride 5 mL in 100 mL Normal Saline IV infusion slowly in 1 hr to start 4 hr after initiation of Insulin infusion

Inj Sodium Bicarbonate (10%) 100 mL IV 2 hrly till pH rises above 7.2

Inj Sod/Pot Phosphate 5 mL in 25 mL of 0.9% saline in IV infusion in 15 min if phosphate is low

Inj Ceftriaxone 1 g IV once

XY Jain
Stamp

Note: Other supportive measures and treatment of precipitating cause must be instituted simultaneously.

CASE SCENARIO 40

A 24-year-old man presented to the emergency department with a five-day history of sore throat, fever, malaise, difficulty in swallowing and hoarseness of voice. On physical examination, temperature 100.4°F, heart rate 100 beats/minute, blood pressure 108/64 mm Hg and respiratory rate 30/minute. Examination of throat showed a grey-white membrane covering the tonsils, uvula, and soft palate. The patient was also noted to have markedly enlarged cervical lymph nodes. Throat and nasopharyngeal swabs culture were positive for *Corynebacterium diphtheriae*. Write a prescription for this patient incorporating all the elements.

Dr XY Jain
MBBS, MD (General Medicine)
Registration no. MPMC 223344
25, Park Street, Gwalior MP
Tel. no. 111222 Email: -------@-----.com

Date: 00.00.0000

Patient's name: Mr X
Age & Sex: 24 years, Male
Address: .... Weight: ....

Diagnosis: Diphtheria

R_x
Inj Procaine Penicillin G 1.2 Million Units IM once daily until the patient can swallow comfortably then switch to
Tab Penicillin V 250 mg orally 6 hrly to complete a 14-day course
Tab Paracetamol 500 mg 6–8 hrly as required for fever
Give first injection after sensitivity test (AST)

XY Jain
Stamp

Alternative Agents

Inj Erythromycin 500 mg IV until the patient can swallow comfortably then, Tab Erythromycin 500 mg orally 6 hrly to complete a 14-day course.

CASE SCENARIO 41

A 29-year-old married lady having one child of 2 year age presents in gynaecology out patient clinic. She wants to avoid pregnancy as she has to appear in a competitive exam after two months. She gave the history of unprotected intercourse two days back. Her date of the last menstrual period was 20 days back. Her blood pressure and other parameters are normal. Write a prescription for this woman.

Dr XY Jain
MBBS, MS (Obstetrics & Gynaecology)
Registration no. MPMC 223344
25, Park Street, Gwalior MP
Tel. no. 111222 Email: -------@-----.com

Date: 00.00.0000

Patient's name: Ms X
Age & Sex: 29 years, Female
Address: .... Weight: ....

Diagnosis: Advised Emergency Contraception

R_X
Tab Levonorgestrel 750 mcg orally stat followed by 750 mcg after 24 hr (total two tablets)

XY Jain
Stamp

Alternative Agents

Tab Levonorgestrel 1.5 mg orally single dose OR

Tab Ethinylestradiol 100 mcg + Levonorgestrel 500 mcg orally stat followed by same dose after 12 hr (total two tablets) OR

Tab Mifepristone 600 mg orally single dose OR

Tab Ulipristal acetate 30 mg orally single dose

CASE SCENARIO 42

A 60-year-old female presents with a fever of 102°F, bodyache, nausea, vomiting, and muscle and joint pains for three days. Her blood test for malaria and typhoid is negative. The platelet count is 70,000/cmm. Her NS 1 antigen test by ELISA is positive. Write a prescription for this patient incorporating all the elements.

Dr XY Jain
MBBS, MD (General Medicine)
Registration no. MPMC 223344
25, Park Street, Gwalior MP
Tel. no. 111222 Email: -------@-----.com

Date: 00.00.0000

Patient's name: Ms X
Age & Sex: 60 years, Female
Address: .... Weight: ....

Diagnosis: Dengue

R_X
Tab Paracetamol 650 mg orally 8 hrly for two days
Tab Ondansetron 4 mg orally as required for vomiting
Cap Omeprazole 40 mg orally once daily for two days
Plenty of fluid orally
Repeat platelet count after 24–48 hrs
Review after 2 days

XY Jain
Stamp

CASE SCENARIO 43

A 12-year-old boy presented of abdominal pain and perianal pruritus, particularly at night for 2 weeks. His abdominal pain was localized to the left upper quadrant and was sharp in nature. Bowel sounds were present on auscultation. An application of clear cellulose acetate tape to the perianal region revealed adult worms and eggs which were identified as *Enterobius vermicularis* or pinworm. Write a prescription for this patient incorporating all the elements.

Dr XY Jain
MBBS, MD (Paediatrics)
Registration no. MPMC 223344
25, Park Street, Gwalior MP
Tel. no. 111222 Email: -------@-----.com

Date: 00.00.0000

Patient's name: Mr X
Age & Sex: 12 years, Male
Address: .... Weight: ....

Diagnosis: *Enterobius vermicularis* Infestation

Rx
Tab Mebendazole 100 mg orally once
Repeat one tab after 2 weeks

XY Jain
Stamp

Other First line Agent

Tab Albendazole 400 mg orally once and repeat after 2 weeks.

CASE SCENARIO 44

A 70-year-old woman presented to the emergency department due to the rapid onset of fever with chills, malaise and a suspected skin infection. On examination, she had temperature of 101°F, respiratory rate of 15 breaths/min, heart rate of 86 beats/min, and blood pressure of 124/72 mmHg. She had a sharply demarcated painful erythema with well-defined indurated margins on her left upper arm. The lesion was warm to the touch, tender, and appeared shiny and swollen. Blood culture was positive for *Streptococcus pyogenes*. Write a prescription for this patient incorporating all the elements.

Dr XY Jain
MBBS, MD (General Medicine)
Registration no. MPMC 223344
25, Park Street, Gwalior MP
Tel. no. 111222 Email: -------@-----.com

Date: 00.00.0000

Patient's name: Ms X
Age & Sex: 70 years, Female
Address: .... Weight: ....

Diagnosis: Erysipelas

R_x
Tab Penicillin V 500 mg orally 6 hrly for 7 days
Tab Paracetamol 500 mg orally 6–8 hrly as required for fever

XY Jain
Stamp

Alternative Agents

Tab Cephlexin 500 mg orally 6 hrly for 7 days OR
Tab Clindamycin 600 mg 12 hrly for 7 days OR
Tab Erythromycin 500 mg 6 hrly for 7 days OR
Cap Amoxicillin 500 mg orally 8 hrly for 7 days

CASE SCENARIO 45

A 62-year-old male patient presented with episodic fever, pain and swelling in the scrotum and gross swelling of his right lower limb for 3 months. Physical examination revealed massive oedema in the right lower limb with non-pitting oedema and skin thickening. Hydrocele was also present. There were 2–3 palpable, non-tender lymph nodes in the right inguinal region. The systemic examination was normal. Haematological investigations were completely normal. A night blood smear examination with Giemsa stain confirmed Bancroftian filariasis. Write a prescription for this patient incorporating all the elements.

Dr XY Jain
MBBS, MD (General Medicine)
Registration no. MPMC 223344
25, Park Street, Gwalior MP
Tel. no. 111222 Email: -------@-----.com

Date: 00.00.0000

Patient's name: Mr X
Age & Sex: 62 years, Male
Address: .... Weight: ....

Diagnosis: Filariasis

R_x
Tab Diethylcarbamazine 100mg 8 hrly for 21 days
Tab Paracetamol 500 mg orally 6-8 hrly for fever

XY Jain
Stamp

CASE SCENARIO 46

A 25-year-old male was brought to the emergency department by his brother. The patient was playing a football game when suddenly the patient fell to the ground and appeared to lose consciousness. His body stiffened with arms and legs extended. He suddenly let out a shrill cry and appeared to stop breathing for about 10 seconds followed by a series of violent, rhythmic, muscle contractions accompanied by hyperventilation and rolling eyes. The jerking movements progressively became less intense until they stopped altogether. The entire episode lasted approximately 3–4 minutes. The patient woke up confused with no recall of the attack but he complained of a headache and extremely sore muscles. Write a prescription for this patient incorporating all the elements.

Dr XY Jain
MBBS, MD (Neurology)
Registration no. MPMC 223344
25, Park Street, Gwalior MP
Tel. no. 111222 Email: -------@-----.com

Date: 00.00.0000

Patient's name: Mr X
Age & Sex: 25 years, Male
Address: .... Weight: ....

Diagnosis: Generalized Tonic Clonic Seizures

R_X
Tab Phenytoin 100 mg orally 8 hrly for 7 days
Tab Clobazam 10 mg orally at bed time for 7 days
Avoid driving vehicles and operating heavy machineries
Review after 7 days for dose escalation

XY Jain
Stamp

Alternative Agents

Tab SodiumValproate 300 mg orally 12 hrly for 7 days OR
Tab Carbamazepine 200 mg orally 12 hrly for 7 days

CASE SCENARIO 47

A 26-year-old male patient presented with severe dysuria and burning sensation during urination with purulent discharge for 4 days. On physical examination, vital signs showed: Blood pressure 110/80 mm Hg, pulse 78 bpm, and temperature 99.6°F. His systemic examination was normal except for spontaneous discharge of pus from the urethral meatus. Gram stain of the urethral discharge showed gram-negative diplococci. Culture of urethral swab was positive for *Neisseria gonorrhoeae*. Write a prescription for this patient incorporating all the elements.

Dr XY Jain
MBBS, MD (Skin & VD)
Registration no. MPMC 223344
25, Park Street, Gwalior MP
Tel. no. 111222 Email: -------@-----.com

Date: 00.00.0000

Patient's name: Mr X
Age & Sex: 26 years, Male
Address: .... Weight: ....

Diagnosis: Gonorrhoea

R_x
Inj Ceftriaxone 250 mg IM single dose
Tab Azithromycin 1g orally single dose
Tab Paracetamol 500 mg orally 6–8 hrly as required for fever

XY Jain
Stamp

Alternative Regimens

Tab Cefixime 400 mg orally single dose + Tab Azithromycin 1 g orally single dose OR
Inj Cefotaxime 500 mg IM single dose + Tab Azithromycin 1 g orally single dose OR
Cap Doxycycline 100 mg orally 12 hrly for 7 days

CASE SCENARIO 48

A 19-year-old unmarried girl complains of pain in the lower abdomen, back and thigh with fatigue every month during periods for the last 2 years. Pain starts 1 or 2 days before periods every month and disappears after three days. Pain is very severe at times. Write a prescription for this patient incorporating all the elements.

Dr XY Jain
MBBS, MS (Obst & Gynae)
Registration no. MPMC 223344
25, Park Street, Gwalior MP
Tel. no. 111222 Email: -------@-----.com

Date: 00.00.0000

Patient's name: Ms X
Age & Sex: 19 years, Female
Address: .... Weight: ....

Diagnosis: Dysmenorrhoea

R_X
Tab Ibuprofen 200 mg orally 6 hrly after meals for five days
Follow up after 5 days

XY Jain
Stamp

Alternative Agents

Tab Mefenamic acid 500 mg orally initially then 250 mg 6 hrly for five days OR
Tab Naproxen 500 mg initially orally then 250 mg orally 12 hrly for five days OR
Tab Etoricoxib 40 mg orally once a day for five days

CASE SCENARIO 49

A 38-year-old man presented with a two-month history of a painless ulcerated lesion on the penis. The patient reported painless nodule that slowly evolved to red ulcerated lesion over 1 month. Physical examination revealed a 1 cm painless ulcer with rolled edges. The base of the ulcer was irregular and beefy-red with friable base of granulation tissue. Inguinal lymph nodes were not palpable. The rest of the physical examination and routine blood and urine tests were normal. A serologic test for syphilis was nonreactive. A biopsy was performed which showed many Donovan bodies. Write a prescription for this patient incorporating all the elements.

Dr XY Jain
MBBS, MD (Skin & VD)
Registration no. MPMC 223344
25, Park Street, Gwalior MP
Tel. no. 111222 Email: -------@-----.com

Date: 00.00.0000

Patient's name: Mr X
Age & Sex: 38 years, Male
Address: .... Weight: ....

Diagnosis: Granuloma Inguinale

Rx
Tab Azithromycin 1 g orally on day 1 followed by 500 mg daily for 7 days

XY Jain
Stamp

Alternative Agents

Tab Trimethoprim/Sulfamethoxazole 160/800 mg orally 12 hrly for 14 days OR
Cap Doxycycline 100 mg orally 12 hrly for 14 days OR
Tab Erythromycin 500 mg orally 6 hrly for 14 days (in pregnant women) OR
Cap Tetracycline 500 mg orally 6 hrly for 14 days OR
Tab Ciprofloxacin 750 mg orally 12 hrly for 14 days

CASE SCENARIO 50

A 54-year-old woman presented to a district hospital with a 3-week history of breathlessness, productive cough, weight loss and lethargy. There was no history of chest pain, wheeze or hemoptysis. She had been recently treated with levofloxacin for a lower respiratory tract infection. On examination, her temperature 100.6°F, with heart rate 110/min and BP 108/64 mm Hg. Auscultation of chest revealed bilateral basal crackles. X-ray chest revealed bilateral basal consolidation. Blood cultures showed growth of gram-negative bacilli—*Haemophilus influenzae*. Write a prescription for this patient incorporating all the elements.

Dr XY Jain
MBBS, MD (General Medicine)
Registration no. MPMC 223344
25, Park Street, Gwalior MP
Tel. no. 111222 Email: -------@-----.com

Date: 00.00.0000

Patient's name: Ms X
Age & Sex: 54 years, Female
Address: .... Weight: ....

Diagnosis: *H. influenzae* Pneumonia

R_X
Cap Amoxicillin 500 mg orally 8 hrly for 10 days
Tab Paracetamol 500 mg orally 6–8 hrly as required for fever

XY Jain
Stamp

Alternatives Agents

Tab Azithromycin 500 mg orally once on day 1 followed by 250 mg daily for 4 days OR
Tab Cefuroxime Axetil 500 mg orally 12 hrly for 7 days OR
Tab Ciprofloxacin 500 mg orally 12 hrly for 7 days OR
Tab Levofloxacin 750 mg orally once daily for 7 days OR
Tab Moxifloxacin 400 mg orally once daily for 7 days OR
Tab Trimethoprim/Sulfamethoxazole (160/800 mg) orally 12 hrly for 7 days OR
Tab Doxycycline 100 mg orally 12 hrly for 7 days

CASE SCENARIO 51

A 27-year-old male reported to the department of dermatology with a complaint of ulcers on upper lip associated with pain, itching and burning for 3 days. Medical history revealed that he was suffering from fever and generalized weakness prior to the ulcerations. On general physical examination, all the vital signs were within normal limits. On extraoral examination, submandibular lymph nodes were palpable both on the left and right sides which were mobile, tender and soft in consistency. Intraoral examination revealed multiple vesicles and shallow ulcers measuring less than 0.5 cm on lower labial mucosa surrounded by an erythematous area. Write a prescription for this patient incorporating all the elements.

Dr XY Jain
MBBS, MD (General Medicine)
Registration no. MPMC 223344
25, Park Street, Gwalior MP
Tel. no. 111222 Email: -------@-----.com

Date: 00.00.0000

Patient's name: Mr X
Age & Sex: 27 years, Male
Address: .... Weight: ....

Diagnosis: Herpes Simplex

R_x
Tab Acyclovir 200 mg orally 5 times daily for 5 days
Penciclovir cream 1% apply locally 2 hrly for 5 days
Tab Paracetamol 500 mg orally 6–8 hrly as required for pain

XY Jain
Stamp

Alternative Agents

Tab Famciclovir 250 mg orally 8 hrly for 7 days OR
Tab Valacyclovir 1000 mg orally12 hrly for 7 days

CASE SCENARIO 52

A 45-year-old businessman, presents with loose, watery stools, abdominal cramping, sweats, fevers and poor appetite for 2 months. He also lost 12 kg weight. He gave a history of frequent business trips to West Africa during the last five year. A month before consulting this clinic, he was treated in Africa for a soft chancre. Three weeks later he developed flu-like symptoms associated with splenomegaly and lymphadenopathy. Several antibiotic courses and malaria treatment had already been prescribed in Western Africa. When seen in this clinic, he was in an unchanged clinical condition and was severely ill. On examination, his temperature 102.4°F, pulse 94/min, respiratory rate 18/min and blood pressure 122/80 mm Hg. Laboratory tests showed anaemia and a CD4 count of 100 cells/mm^3. Serology revealed a positive HIV-1 ELISA and Western blot tests. Write a prescription for this patient incorporating all the elements.

Dr XY Jain
MBBS, MD (General Medicine)
Registration no. MPMC 223344
25, Park Street, Gwalior MP
Tel. no. 111222 Email: -------@-----.com

Date: 00.00.0000

Patient's name: Mr X
Age & Sex: 45 years, Male
Address: .... Weight: ....

Diagnosis: Human Immunodeficiency Virus Infection

R_x
Tab Tenofovir 300 mg orally once daily for 1 month
Tab Lamivudine 300 mg orally once daily for 1 month
Tab Dolutegravir 50 mg once daily for 1 month
Tab Paracetamol 500 mg orally 6–8 hrly as required for fever
Refill 11

XY Jain
Stamp

Alternative Regimen

Tab Tenofovir 300 mg orally once daily for 1 month +
Tab Lamivudine 300 mg orally once daily for 1 month +
Tab Efavirenz 600 mg orally once daily for 1 month

CASE SCENARIO 53

A 58-year-old man with hypertension and type II diabetes is taking an angiotensin-converting enzyme (ACE) inhibitor-thiazide diuretic combination for his hypertension and metformin for his diabetes. His blood pressure and diabetes are under control and renal function and liver function tests are normal. His lipid profile shows total cholesterol 260 mg/dL, LDL 190 mg/dL, triglycerides 130 mg/dL and high density lipoprotein 38 mg/dL. To reduce his risk of developing coronary artery disease, a lipid-lowering drug is to be added to his present treatment regimen. Write a prescription for this patient incorporating all the elements.

Dr XY Jain
MBBS, MD (General Medicine)
Registration no. MPMC 223344
25, Park Street, Gwalior MP
Tel. no. 111222 Email: -------@-----.com

Date: 00.00.0000

Patient's name: Mr X
Age & Sex: 58 years, Male
Address: .... Weight: ....

Diagnosis: Hypercholesterolemia

R_x
Tab Atorvastatin 20 mg orally once daily for 1 month
Review after one month

XY Jain
Stamp

Alternative Agents

Tab Lovastatin 20–40 mg orally once daily for 1 month OR
Tab Pravastatin 40–80 mg orally once daily for 1 month OR
Tab Simvastatin 20–40 mg orally once daily for 1 month OR
Tab Fluvastatin 20–40 mg orally once daily for 1 month OR
Tab Rosuvastatin 5–20 mg orally once daily for 1 month OR
Tab Pitavastatin 1–2 mg orally once daily for 1 month

CASE SCENARIO 54

A 35-year-old male patient presents to a gastroenterologist with the complaint of burning pain in the chest for one month. The pain is worst after 2–3 hrs of food intake and heartburn awakens him often at night. The patient had tried antacids but was in partial relief. There are no complaints of pain in the abdomen, vomiting or passing of black stool. Upper gastrointestinal endoscopy reveals erosions in the lower oesophagus. Write a prescription for this patient incorporating all the elements.

Dr XY Jain
MBBS, MD (General Medicine)
Registration no. MPMC 223344
25, Park Street, Gwalior MP
Tel. no. 111222 Email: -------@-----.com

Date: 00.00.0000

Patient's name: Mr X
Age & Sex: 35 years, Male
Address: .... Weight: ....

Diagnosis: Gasroesophageal reflux disease (GERD)

R_x
Cap Omeprazole 20 mg orally once a day on empty stomach in the morning for 7 days
Tab Amisulpiride 20 mg before meals for 7 days
Liq. Sodium alginate gel 2 tsf orally after meals for 7 days
Frequent small non spicy meals
Raise the head end of the bed
Review after 7 days

XY Jain
Stamp

Alternative Agents

Tab Rabeprazole 20 mg orally once a day on empty stomach in the morning for 7 days
OR
Tab Pantoprazole 40 mg orally once a day on empty stomach in the morning for 7 days

CASE SCENARIO 55

A 28-year-old female having 24 weeks of pregnancy attended antenatal clinic with complaints of heaviness in head for 4 days. On examination, her BP was 150/90 mm Hg with oedema over feet. Her Hb level was 12 g/dL. Per abdominal examination was suggestive of 24 weeks of pregnancy. Write a prescription for this patient incorporating all the elements.

Dr XY Jain
MBBS, MD (General Medicine)
Registration no. MPMC 223344
25, Park Street, Gwalior MP
Tel. no. 111222 Email: -------@-----.com

Date: 00.00.0000

Patient's name: Ms X
Age & Sex: 28 years, Female
Address: .... Weight: ....

Diagnosis: Hypertension in Pregnancy

R_x
Tab Methyldopa 250 mg orally 8 hrly for 7 days
Review after 7 days

XY Jain
Stamp

Alternative Agents

Tab Labetalol 100 mg orally 12 hrly for 7 days OR
Tab Nifedipine 30 mg orally once daily for 7 days

CASE SCENARIO 56

A 32-year-old male patient of hypertension was taking tablet Metoprolol since one year and was alright. He suffered from peptic ulcer and was treated for that 3 months back. He has not taken metoprolol for last three months. He was brought to ICU with severe headache, swelling over limbs and reduced urine output. On examination, his blood pressure 200/120 mm Hg, blood urea 44 mg/dL, serum creatinine 1.9 mg/dL and random blood sugar 140 mg/dL. Patient was admitted in medicine ICU. Write a prescription for this patient.

Dr XY Jain
MBBS, MD (General Medicine)
Registration no. MPMC 223344
25, Park Street, Gwalior MP
Tel. no. 111222 Email: -------@-----.com

Date: 00.00.0000

Patient's name: Mr X
Age & Sex: 32 years, Male
Address: .... Weight: ....

Diagnosis: Hypertensive Emergency

R_x

Inj Labetalol 20 mg IV over 2 min then 40 mg every 10 min until BP is reduced by 25% then switch over to oral drugs
(Max dose 300 mg in 24 hr)

XY Jain
Stamp

Alternative Agents

Inj Nicardipine 5 mg/hr IV, titrate by 2.5 mg/hr at 5–10 min interval (Max. 15 mg/hr) OR

Inj Nitroglycerine 5 mcg/min IV, titrate by 5 mcg/min at 5 min interval up to 20 mcg/min OR

Inj Esmolol 500 mcg/kg IV over 1 min, then 50–300 mcg/kg/min OR

Inj Sodium Nitroprusside 0.25–10 mcg/kg/min IV

CASE SCENARIO 57

A 35-year-old male complained of nervousness, weakness, weight loss, heat intolerance and occasional palpitations for the past 3 months. On examination, his pulse was 110/minute and BP was 136/70 mm of Hg. There were tremors of outstretched fingers and lid lag was present. He had diffuse, nontender, smooth enlargement of the thyroid. His thyroid-stimulating hormone level (TSH) was low and T4 level was elevated. Write a prescription for this patient incorporating all the elements.

Dr XY Jain
MBBS, MD (General Medicine)
Registration no. MPMC 223344
25, Park Street, Gwalior MP
Tel. no. 111222 Email: -------@-----.com

Date: 00.00.0000

Patient's name: Mr X
Age & Sex: 35 years, Male
Address: .... Weight: ....

Diagnosis: Hyperthyroidism

R_x
Tab Carbimazole 15 mg orally 8 hrly for 15 days
Refill: 5
Repeat TSH estimation after 3 months for dose adjustment

XY Jain
Stamp

Alternative Agents

If hyperthyroidism in pregnancy
Tab Propylthiouracil 100–150 mg orally 8 hrly till delivery

CASE SCENARIO 58

A 65-year-old, Type II diabetic patient was maintained on insulin for last ten year. His blood sugar was well controlled and his treating physician was satisfied. One evening this patient went to gym after taking insulin and escaped meals. He was brought to the casualty department in semiconscious state. His blood sugar level was 30 mg/dL. Patient was admitted in casualty ward. Write a prescription for this patient.

Dr XY Jain
MBBS, MD (General Medicine)
Registration no. MPMC 223344
25, Park Street, Gwalior MP
Tel. no. 111222 Email: -------@-----.com

Date: 00.00.0000

Patient's name: Mr X
Age & Sex: 65 years, Male
Address: .... Weight: ....

Diagnosis: Hypoglycemia

R_x
Inj Dextrose (50%) 50 mL IV bolus in 3–5 min

XY Jain
Stamp

Alternative Agents

Inj Glucagon 1 mg SC or IM or IV stat

CASE SCENARIO 59

A 45-year-old female presents with complaints of progressive weight gain of 4 kilograms in 6 months, fatigue, slight memory loss, slow speech, deepening of her voice, dry skin, constipation, and cold intolerance. On examination, her blood pressure is 124/82 mm Hg and heart rate is 70/minute. Her thyroid gland feels diffusely enlarged, nontender and firm in consistency. Her thyroid-stimulating hormone level (TSH) is elevated, and T4 level is reduced. Patient was admitted in medicine ward. Write a prescription for this patient incorporating all the elements.

Dr XY Jain
MBBS, MD (General Medicine)
Registration no. MPMC 223344
25, Park Street, Gwalior MP
Tel. no. 111222 Email: -------@-----.com

Date: 00.00.0000

Patient's name: Ms X
Age & Sex: 45 years, Female
Address: .... Weight: ....

Diagnosis: Hypothyroidism

R_X
Tab Levothyroxine 50 mcg orally once daily 30 min before breakfast for 4 weeks.
Refils: 2
Repeat TSH after 12 weeks for dose adjustment

XY Jain
Stamp

CASE SCENARIO 60

A 62-year-old male with prior medical history of hypertension, presented to the emergency department of a tertiary care hospital with symptoms of rigors, chills, fever, weakness and lower extremity edema for two weeks. On examination, his temperature was 100.4°F, pulse rate was 94/minute, respiratory rate was 24/minute, blood pressure was 104/56 mm Hg and oxygen saturation on room air was 90%. Bilateral lower extremity edema was present with erythema. ECG was normal. A transthoracic echocardiogram was performed which revealed mitral valve vegetations, minimal mitral valve regurgitation, and a normal ejection fraction of 55%. Patient was admitted in medicine ward. Blood culture was positive for *Enterococcus faecalis*. Write a prescription for this patient incorporating all the elements.

Dr XY Jain
MBBS, MD (General Medicine)
Registration no. MPMC 223344
25, Park Street, Gwalior MP
Tel. no. 111222 Email: -------@-----.com

Date: 00.00.0000

Patient's name: Mr X
Age & Sex: 62 years, Male
Address: .... Weight: ....

Diagnosis: Infective Endocarditis

R_x
Inj Penicillin G 4 Million Units IV 4 hrly for 2 weeks
Inj Gentamicin 60 mg IV 8 hrly for 2 weeks
Tab Paracetamol 500 mg orally 6–8 hrly as required for fever
Inj Penicillin to be started after sensitivity test
Review after 2 weeks
Refills: 2

XY Jain
Stamp

Alternative Agents to Penicillin G

Inj Ampicillin 2 g IV 4 hrly for 2 weeks OR
Inj Ceftriaxone 2 g IV 12 hrly for 2 weeks OR
Inj Amoxyclav 1.2 g IV 6 hrly for 2 weeks OR
Inj Vancomycin 1 g IV 12 hrly for 2 weeks

CASE SCENARIO 61

A 60-year-old man presents to his family physician with a complaint of persistent insomnia for approximately 4 months. Initially, he only had difficulty staying asleep but now he has frequent nocturnal awakenings. He wakes up two or more times per night and on most nights has difficulty falling asleep. Over the past two months, daytime sleepiness and fatigue have increased in severity associated with diminished energy, poor concentration, memory impairment, irritability and depressed or anxious mood. His physical examination is normal. Write a prescription for this patient incorporating all the elements.

Dr XY Jain
MBBS, MD (General Medicine)
Registration no. MPMC 223344
25, Park Street, Gwalior MP
Tel. no. 111222 Email: -------@-----.com

Date: 00.00.0000

Patient's name: Mr X
Age & Sex: 60 years, Male
Address: .... Weight: ....

Diagnosis: Insomnia

R_x
Tab Zopiclone 7.5 mg orally once at bed time for 7 days
Review after 7 days

XY Jain
Stamp

Alternative Agents

Tab Eszopiclone 3 mg orally once at bed time for 7 days OR
Tab Zolpidem 10 mg orally once at bed time for 7 days OR
Tab Nitrazepam 5 mg orally once at bed timefor 7 days OR
Tab Zaleplon 10 mg orally once at bed time for 7 days

CASE SCENARIO 62

A 30-year-old woman presented to her family physician with the complaints of generalized weakness, easy fatigability, palpitations, and dyspnoea on exertion. She stated that these symptoms had started about 3 months ago and had become progressively worse over the past 2 weeks. The patient has no history of menorrhagia or overt evidence of bleeding from any site. Physical examination revealed a smooth tongue, brittle nails, spooning of nails and pale conjunctiva. Her vitals were as follows: Blood pressure 128/76 mm Hg, pulse 108 bpm, respirations 24/min, body temperature 97.7°F. Stools were negative for occult blood. Complete blood count showed Hg 7.1 gm/dL with a low ferritin level. Write a prescription for this patient incorporating all the elements.

Dr XY Jain
MBBS, MD (General Medicine)
Registration no. MPMC 223344
25, Park Street, Gwalior MP
Tel. no. 111222 Email: -------@-----.com

Date: 00.00.0000

Patient's name: Ms X
Age & Sex: 30 years, Female
Address: .... Weight: ....

Diagnosis: Iron Deficiency Anaemia

R_X
Tab Ferrous Sulfate 200 mg orally 8 hrly after meals for 1 month
Oral iron makes the stool black
Review after 1 month

XY Jain
Stamp

Alternative Agents

Tab Ferrous Fumarate 200 mg orally 8 hrly for 1 month OR
Tab Ferrous Gluconate 300 mg orally 8 hrly for 1 month

CASE SCENARIO 63

A 63-year-old man weighing 70 kg was brought to ICU with breathlessness and swelling over feet for 7 days. He gave history of stent placement in left coronary artery five year back during angiography for unstable angina and was well controlled. On examination, his BP was 160/100 mm Hg. On auscultation, basal crepitations were present on both sides of lungs. Urine output was 800 mL in 24 hr. Blood urea was 30 mg/dL. His echocardiography revealed ejection fraction below normal. Patient was admitted in medicine ICU. Write a prescription for this patient.

Dr XY Jain
MBBS, MD (General Medicine)
Registration no. MPMC 223344
25, Park Street, Gwalior MP
Tel. no. 111222 Email: -------@-----.com

Date: 00.00.0000

Patient's name: Mr X
Age & Sex: 63 years, Male
Weight: 73 kg
Address: ....

Diagnosis: Left Ventricular Failure

R_x
Immediate hospitalization in ICU
Oxygen inhalation, if saturation is less than 90%
Inj Furosemide 40 mg IV stat
Inj Dopamine 50 mcg /min IV infusion
Tab Isosorbide Dinitrate 20 mg orally 12 hrly
Pot Chloride solution 5 mL orally with 100 mL of water 12 hrly.
Review after 24 hr

XY Jain
Stamp

CASE SCENARIO 64

A 45-year-old woman presented to an emergency department with a three-day history of fever, chills, headache, nausea, vomiting, abdominal pain, conjunctival congestion, arthralgia, myalgia, and loss of appetite. She gave history of a recent rat bite for which she received tetanus toxoid and wound care at a nearby clinic. Her complete blood count showed anemia, leukocytosis with neutrophilia and thrombocytopenia. Clinical examination recorded a temperature of 104°F, blood pressure of 118/76 mm Hg, heart rate of 104 beats/minute and respiratory rate of 16/minute. On abdominal palpation splenomegaly was present. Leptospiral strip test for IgM antibodies was positive. Patient was admitted in medicine ward. Write a prescription for this patient incorporating all the elements.

Dr XY Jain
MBBS, MD (General Medicine)
Registration no. MPMC 223344
25, Park Street, Gwalior MP
Tel. no. 111222 Email: -------@-----.com

Date: 00.00.0000

Patient's name: Ms X
Age & Sex: 45 years, Female
Address: .... Weight: ....

Diagnosis: Leptospirosis

R_x

Inj Penicillin G 1.5 Million Units IV 6 hrly till required then switch to Tab Penicillin V 500 mg four times daily until 10 days

Tab Paracetamol 500 mg orally 6–8 hrly as required for fever

Inj Penicillin to be started after sensitivity test

XY Jain
Stamp

Alternative Agents to Penicillin G

Inj Ceftriaxone 1 g IV once daily till required OR

Inj Cefotaxime 1 g IV 6 hrly till required

Alternative Agents to Penicillin V

Cap/Tab Amoxicillin 500 mg 8 hrly to complete 10 days of therapy.

CASE SCENARIO 65

A 48-year-old male presented with a 5-day history of fever, headache, nausea and diarrhoea. He had up to 15 episodes of diarrhea in the last 24 hours. The patient revealed that he frequently attended parties and enjoyed fruits, salads, and cheese. On physical examination, his temperature 101.4°F, blood pressure 96/60 mm Hg, and pulse 120 per minute. CBC showed leukocytosis. CT of abdomen revealed enteritis and colitis of the descending sigmoid colon. The patient's blood culture was positive for *Listeria monocytogenes*. Patient was admitted in medicine ward. Write a prescription for this patient incorporating all the elements.

Dr XY Jain
MBBS, MD (General Medicine)
Registration no. MPMC 223344
25, Park Street, Gwalior MP
Tel. no. 111222 Email: -------@-----.com

Date: 00.00.0000

Patient's name: Mr X
Age & Sex: 48 years, Male
Address: .... Weight: ....

Diagnosis: Listeriosis

R_x
Inj Ampicillin 2 g IV 6 hrly for 14 days
Inj Gentamicin 240 mg IV once daily for 14 days
Tab Paracetamol 500 mg orally 6–8 hrly as required for fever

XY Jain
Stamp

In Penicillin Allergic Patients

Inj Trimethoprim/Sulfamethoxazole (10–20 mg/kg of the Trimethoprim component IV 6 hrly) orally for 14 days.

CASE SCENARIO 66

A 50-year-old male presented with a 5-day history of extreme headaches, fever with chills, generalized joint pain and sudden appearance of a painful red papule on back of his right thigh, which was increasing progressively. He gave a history of visit to the nearby forest a few days before the appearance of the lesion. On examination, there was an erythematous annular plaque on back of the right thigh approximately 5 centimeter in diameter with a central brownish fluid filled blister. Serology for *Borrelia burgdorferi* antigen was done with enzyme-immunoassay technique. IgM was raised, whereas IgG was found to be normal. Write a prescription for this patient incorporating all the elements.

Dr XY Jain
MBBS, MD (General Medicine)
Registration no. MPMC 223344
25, Park Street, Gwalior MP
Tel. no. 111222 Email: -------@-----.com

Date: 00.00.0000

Patient's name: Mr X
Age & Sex: 50 years, Male
Address: .... Weight: ....

Diagnosis: Lyme Disease

R_x
Cap Doxycycline 100 mg orally 12 hrly on empty stomach for 14 days
Tab Paracetamol 500 mg orally 6–8 hrly as required for fever
Avoid iron, milk and dairy products with the drug

XY Jain
Stamp

Alternative Agents

Cap Amoxicillin 500 mg orally 8 hrly for 21 days OR
Tab Cefuroxime Axetil 500 mg orally 12 hrly for 21 days OR
Tab Erythromycin 250 mg orally 6 hrly for 21 days

CASE SCENARIO 67

A 40-year-old man presented at STD clinic with a painful penile ulcer, mild fever and general malaise. On physical examination, the temperature was 100.4 °F with a marked swelling in the right groin which was firm, fluctuant, and slightly tender. The penile ulcer was 2.5 cm in diameter. The bottom of the ulcer was red and showed some purulent exudates. Edges of the ulcer were elevated and round. PCR was done in the biopsy of the penis lesion which was positive for *Chlamydia trachomatis*. Serology for *C. trachomatis* showed relatively high levels of IgA and IgG. Write a prescription for this patient incorporating all the elements.

Dr XY Jain
MBBS, MD (Skin & VD)
Registration no. MPMC 223344
25, Park Street, Gwalior MP
Tel. no. 111222 Email: -------@-----.com

Date: 00.00.0000

Patient's name: Mr X
Age & Sex: 40 years, Male
Address: .... Weight: ....

Diagnosis: Lymphogranuloma Venereum

R_x
Cap Doxycycline 100 mg orally 12 hrly for 21 days
Tab Paracetamol 500 mg orally 6–8 hrly as required for fever

XY Jain
Stamp

Alternative Agents

Tab Erythromycin 500 mg orally 6 hrly for 21 days OR
Tab Azithromycin 1 g orally once weekly for 3 weeks OR
Cap Tetracycline 500 mg orally 6 hrly for 21 days OR
Tab Moxifloxacin 400 mg orally once daily for 21 days

CASE SCENARIO 68

A 55-year-old male presents with fever with chills, rigors, vomiting and headache for 5 days. He has recently came from an area where chloroquine resistant falciparum malaria is prevalent. Per abdominal examination reveals splenomegaly. Complete blood count shows Hb 7.5 g/dL. Peripheral blood smear showed *P. falciparum*. Write a prescription for this patient.

Dr XY Jain
MBBS, MD (General Medicine)
Registration no. MPMC 223344
25, Park Street, Gwalior MP
Tel. no. 111222 Email: -------@-----.com

Date: 00.00.0000

Patient's name: Mr X
Age & Sex: 55 years, Male
Address: .... Weight: ....

Diagnosis: Malaria—*P. falciparum* (Uncomplicated)

R_x
Tab Artemether 80 mg + Lumefantrine 480 mg orally 12 hrly for 3 days
Tab Paracetamol 500 mg orally 6–8 hrly as required for fever
Tab Metoclopramide 10 mg orally 8 hrly before meals as required for vomiting

XY Jain
Stamp

Alternative Agents

Tab Artesunate 100 mg orally 12 hrly for 3 days +
Tab Mefloquine 750 mg orally stat followed by 500 mg after 12 hr OR
Tab Artesunate 100 mg orally 12 hrly for 3 days +
Tab Sulfadoxine + Pyrimethamine 1500 mg/75 mg orally single dose OR
Tab Quinine 600 mg orally 8 hrly for 7 days +
Cap Doxycycline 100 mg orally once for 7 days OR
Tab Clindamycin 600 mg orally 12 hrly for 7 days OR
Cap Tetracycline 250 mg orally 6 hrly for 7 days

CASE SCENARIO 69

A 35-year-old male presented to the hospital with a 5-day history of intermittent fever with chills and rigors, headache, nausea and vomiting. On examination, his temperature was 102°F and heart rate was 112/minute. Mild tenderness in the right hypochondrium with hepatomegaly was also noted. Examination of peripheral blood smears revealed rings and trophozoites typical of the *P. vivax*. The patient was treated with oral chloroquine 10 mg/kg, 10 mg/kg and 5 mg/kg body wt on days 1, 2 and 3 respectively. But the patient remained febrile on completion of chloroquine therapy, therefore peripheral blood smear examination was repeated which continued to show *P. vivax*. Write a prescription for this patient incorporating all the elements.

Dr XY Jain
MBBS, MD (General Medicine)
Registration no. MPMC 223344
25, Park Street, Gwalior MP
Tel. no. 111222 Email: -------@-----.com

Date: 00.00.0000

Patient's name: Mr X
Age & Sex: 35 years, Male
Address: .... Weight: ....

Diagnosis: Malaria—*P. vivax* (Chloroquine Resistant)

R_x
Tab Mefloquine 750 mg orally once and 500 mg after 12 hr
Tab Primaquine 15 mg orally once daily for 14 days.
Tab Paracetamol 500 mg orally 6–8 hrly as required for fever
Tab Metoclopramide 10 mg orally 8 hrly before meals as required for vomiting

XY Jain
Stamp

Alternative Agents to Mefloquin

Tab Sulphadoxine + Pyrimethamine (1500 mg/75) mg orally once OR
Tab Quinine 600 mg orally 8 hrly for 7 days +
Cap Doxycycline 100 mg orally once for 7 days OR
Tab Clindamycin 600 mg orally 12 hrly for 7 days OR
Cap Tetracycline 250 mg orally 6 hrly for 7 days

CASE SCENARIO 70

A 34-year-old female presented to the hospital with a 5-day history of intermittent fever with chills, headache, nausea, vomiting, loss of appetite, generalized weakness and body pains. On examination, her temperature was 102°F and heart rate was 112/minute. Mild tenderness in the right hypochondrium with hepatomegaly was also noted. Examination of peripheral blood smears revealed rings and trophozoites typical of the *P. vivax*. Write a prescription for this patient incorporating all the elements.

Dr XY Jain
MBBS, MD (General Medicine)
Registration no. MPMC 223344
25, Park Street, Gwalior MP
Tel. no. 111222 Email: -------@-----.com

Date: 00.00.0000

Patient's name: Ms X
Age & Sex: 34 years, Female
Address: .... Weight: ....

Diagnosis: Malaria—*P. vivax* (Chloroquine Sensitive)

R_x
Tab Chloroquine phosphate 600 mg base (1g salt) orally once

Followed by
Tab Chloroquine phosphate 300 mg base (500 mg salt) orally after meals at 6, 24 and 48 hours. Followed by:
Tab Primaquine 15 mg orally once daily for 14 days.
Tab Paracetamol 500 mg orally 6–8 hrly as required for fever
Tab Metoclopramide 10 mg orally 8 hrly before meals as required for vomiting
Get test done for G6PD status before starting Primaquine

XY Jain
Stamp

CASE SCENARIO 71

A 45-year-old male, weighing 60 kg, diagnosed with primary tuberculosis was on first line anti-tubercular treatment. The patient did not show improvement in cough, fever and breathlessness after one month of therapy. His sputum for AFB was positive. He was advised CB NAAT test which showed rifampicin resistance. Write a prescription for his patient incorporating all the elements.

Dr XY Jain
MBBS, MD (General Medicine)
Registration no. MPMC 223344
25, Park Street, Gwalior MP
Tel. no. 111222 Email: -------@-----.com

Date: 00.00.0000

Patient's name: Mr X
Age & Sex: 45 years, Male
Weight: 60 kg
Address: ....

Diagnosis: MDR Tuberculosis

R_X
Tab. Isoniazid 900 mg (high dose) orally once daily for 30 days
Tab Ethambutol 1200 mg orally once daily for 30 days
Tab Pyrazinamide 750 mg orally 12 hrly for 30 days
Tab Levofloxacin 500 mg orally once daily for 30 days
Tab Bedaquiline 200 mg orally 12 hrly for 2 weeks and then 200 mg orally once on alternate day from 3rd to 24th week
Tab Clofazimine 100 mg orally once daily for 30 days
Tab Ethionamide 500 mg orally once daily for 30 days
Tab Pyridoxine 50 mg orally once daily for 30 days
Review every month
Get eye examination done before starting Ethambutol
Refills: 3

XY Jain
Stamp

Note: Sputum for AFB will be repeated after 4 months of initial phase treatment. If the sputum is positive continue above treatment for 2 more months. Switch to following continuation phase treatment after 4 months and 6 months for AFB negative and positive cases respectively.

Tab Ethambutol 1200 mg orally once daily for 5 months

Tab Pyrazinamide 750 mg orally 12 hrly for 5 months

Tab Clofazimine 100 mg orally once daily for 5 months

Tab Ethionamide 500 mg orally once daily for 5 months

Alternative Regimen (When Bedaquiline is either not available or not suitable)

Inj Kanamycin 1g IM one daily for 30 days

Tab Isoniazid 900 mg (high dose) orally once daily for 30 days

Tab Ethambutol 1200 mg orally once daily for 30 days

Tab Pyrazinamide 750 mg orally 12 hrly for 30 days

Tab Moxifloxacin 800 mg orally once daily for 30 days

Tab Clofazimine 100 mg orally once daily for 30 days

Tab Ethionamide 500 mg orally once daily for 30 days

Tab Pyridoxine 50 mg orally once daily for 30 days

Review every month

Get eye examination done before starting ethambutol
Refill: 3

Note: Sputum for AFB will be repeated after 4 months of initial phase treatment. If the sputum is positive continue above treatment for 2 more months. Switch to following continuation phase treatment after 4 months and 6 months for AFB negative and positive cases respectively.

Tab Pyrazinamide 750 mg orally 12 hrly for 5 months

Tab Moxifloxacin 800 mg orally once daily for 5 months

Tab Clofazimine 100 mg orally once daily for 5 months

Tab Ethionamide 500 mg orally once daily for 5 months

Tab Pyridoxine 50 mg orally once daily for 5 months

CASE SCENARIO 72

A 55-year-old woman presented to her family physician with the complaints of generalized weakness, easy fatigability, pain in the legs on walking and dyspnoea on exertion. She stated that these symptoms had started about 6 months ago and had become progressively worse over the past 2 months. She also noted recently increased forgetfulness, some pain on her tongue, tingling and numbness of the fingers. The patient has no history of menorrhagia or overt evidence of bleeding from any site. She was a strict vegetarian. Her vitals were normal except for a heart rate of 120 beats/minute. The patient's conjunctiva, oral mucosa, and nail beds were pale, and her tongue was red and painful. Neurological examination disclosed decreased cutaneous pain and vibratory sensation in both the upper and lower extremities. Her hematological investigations revealed haemoglobin 7.2 g/dL, mean corpuscular volume (MCV) 116 fL (normal 80–100), ferritin levels 300 ng/mL (normal 20–250). Write a prescription for this patient incorporating all the elements.

Dr XY Jain
MBBS, MD (General Medicine)
Registration no. MPMC 223344
25, Park Street, Gwalior MP
Tel. no. 111222 Email: -------@-----.com

Date: 00.00.0000

Patient's name: Ms X
Age & Sex: 55 years, Female
Address: .... Weight: ....

Diagnosis: Megaloblastic Anaemia

Rx
Inj Hydroxocobalamin 1 mg IM once weekly for 6 weeks
Once initial correction of the deficiency has occurred, then
Inj Hydroxocobalamin 1 mg IM once every 3 months
Tab Folic acid 10 mg orally once daily for 6 weeks

XY Jain
Stamp

CASE SCENARIO 73

A 51-year-old male presents with a history of severe episodic vertigo spells lasting 30 minutes to several hours accompanied by right sensorineural hearing loss and tinnitus. He states that he has experienced vertigo spells with right-sided tinnitus a few times per month for the last 6 months. Audiogram revealed a severe sensorineural hearing loss at 35.0 dB, with a predominance of low-frequency impairment in the right ear. Write a prescription for this patient incorporating all the elements.

Dr XY Jain
MBBS, MS (ENT)
Registration no. MPMC 223344
25, Park Street, Gwalior MP
Tel. no. 111222 Email: -------@-----.com

Date: 00.00.0000

Patient's name: Mr X
Age & Sex: 51 years, Male
Address: .... Weight: ....

Diagnosis: Meniere's Disease

R_x
Tab Betahistine 16 mg orally 12 hrly for 7 days

XY Jain
Stamp

Alternative Agents

Tab Dimenhydrinate 50 mg orally 8 hrly for 7 days OR
Tab Meclizine 25 mg orally 12 hrly for 7 days OR
Tab Promethazine 25 mg orally 6 hrly for 7 days

CASE SCENARIO 74

A 25-year-old man presented with acute onset of intense headache, fever, nausea, vomiting, photophobia and stiff neck. On admission, the patient's BP was 108/50 mm Hg, pulse rate was 114 bpm and oral temperature was 102.5°F. He was fully conscious and clinically stable. On neurologic examination, nuchal rigidity was present and Kernig and Brudzinski signs were positive. CSF was turbid with predominating polymorphs, decreased glucose concentration and increased protein concentration. Culture of CSF identified the aetiologic organism as *Neisseria meningitidis*. Patient was admitted in medicine ward. Write a prescription for this patient incorporating all the

Dr XY Jain
MBBS, MD (General Medicine)
Registration no. MPMC 223344
25, Park Street, Gwalior MP
Tel. no. 111222 Email: -------@-----.com

Date: 00.00.0000

Patient's name: Mr X
Age & Sex: 25 years, Male
Address: .... Weight: ....

Diagnosis: Meningococcal Meningitis

R_x
Inj Ceftriaxone 2 g IV 12 hrly 10 days

XY Jain
Stamp

elements.

Alternative Agents

Inj. Penicillin G 4 Million Units AST IV 4 hrly for 7 days OR
Inj Cefotaxime 2 g IV 6 hrly for 10 days OR
Inj Ampicillin 2 g IV 4 hrly for 7 days

Note: All close contacts should receive ***chemoprophylaxis*** with:
Tab Rifampin 600 mg orally 12 hrly for 2 days OR
Tab Azithromycin 500 mg orally single dose OR
Tab Ciprofloxacin 500 mg orally single dose OR
Inj Ceftriaxone 250 mg IM single dose

CASE SCENARIO 75

A 30-year-old male weighing 52 kg took about 300 mL of locally made alcohol. He was brought to the emergency department 2 hours later. On examination, the patient was drowsy. His vital signs were BP 128/82 mm Hg, pulse rate 70/min, temperature 98°F, respiratory rate 18/min. Oxygen saturation was 96% on room air. Respiratory and cardiovascular examinations were normal. The neurological evaluation showed evidence of bilateral nystagmus. Both pupils were dilated with sluggish light reflexes. Arterial blood gas analysis revealed severe metabolic acidosis with pH 6.9 and bicarbonate level being 5 mEq/L. Patient was admitted in medicine ward. Write a prescription for this patient incorporating all the elements.

Dr XY Jain
MBBS, MD (General Medicine)
Registration no. MPMC 223344
25, Park Street, Gwalior MP
Tel. no. 111222 Email: -------@-----.com

Date: 00.00.0000

Patient's name: Mr X
Age & Sex: 30 years, Male
Weight: 52 kg
Address: ....

Diagnosis: Methanol Poisoning

R_X
Inj Ethyl Alcohol (10%) IV 50 mL in 5% dextrose slowly over one h
Followed by 7.5 mL/hr till serum methanol falls below 20 mg/dL
Inj Fomepizole 0.75 mL IV followed by 0.5 mL 12 hrly till serum methanol falls below 20 mg/dL
Inj Sodium Bicarbonate (10%) 100 mL IV 2 hrly till pH rises above 7.2

XY Jain
Stamp

CASE SCENARIO 76

A 28-year-old woman presented to the neurology clinic with a 3-month history of left-sided pulsatile headaches occurring twice a month, each episode lasting 2–3 days. The patient told that her headaches were usually preceded by lightheadedness and unformed flashes of the light. Her headaches were always unilateral and were associated with nausea, vomiting, and photophobia. She also reported sensitivity to light and noise during these episodes. General physical and neurologic examinations were normal. Write a prescription for this patient incorporating all the elements.

Dr XY Jain
MBBS, MD (General Medicine)
Registration no. MPMC 223344
25, Park Street, Gwalior MP
Tel. no. 111222 Email: -------@-----.com

Date: 00.00.0000

Patient's name: Ms X
Age & Sex: 28 years, Female
Address: .... Weight: ....

Diagnosis: Migraine

R_x
Tab Paracetamol 500 mg orally 6 hrly for 3 days
Tab Naratriptan 2.5 mg orally at the onset, may be repeated once after 4 hr then 2.5 mg orally once daily for 3 days
Tab Metoclopramide 10 mg orally 8 hrly as required for vomiting
Review after 3 days

XY Jain
Stamp

Alternative Agents to Paracetamol

Tab Naproxen 250 mg orally 12 hrly as required for pain OR
Tab Ibuprofen 400 mg orally 8 hrly as required for pain

Alternative Agents to Naratriptan

Tab Rizatriptan 5 mg orally at onset, may repeat after 2 hr OR
Tab Sumatriptan 50 mg orally at onset, may repeat after 2 hr OR
Tab Frovatriptan 2.5 mg orally at onset, may repeat after 2 hr OR
Tab Zolmitriptan 2.5 mg orally at onset, may repeat after 2 hr

CASE SCENARIO 77

A 55-year-old male patient came to medical OPD with complaints of headache, dizziness and fatigue off and on for one month. His headache was not relieved by taking paracetamol. On examination, his BP was 150/90 mm Hg when measured consequently for 3 days. His random blood sugar was 130 mg/dL. Blood urea was 20 mg/dL. Write a prescription for this patient incorporating all the elements.

Dr XY Jain
MBBS, MD (General Medicine)
Registration no. MPMC 223344
25, Park Street, Gwalior MP
Tel. no. 111222 Email: -------@-----.com

Date: 00.00.0000

Patient's name: Mr X
Age & Sex: 55 years, Male
Address: .... Weight: ....

Diagnosis: Mild Hypertension

R_x
Tab Chlorthalidone 12.5 mg orally once daily for 7 days
Salt restriction
Regular brisk walking for at least 30 min per day
Review after 7 days

XY Jain
Stamp

Alternative Agents

Tab Lisinopril 5 mg orally once daily for 7 days OR
Tab Telmisartan 40 mg orally once daily for 7 days OR
Tab Amlodipine 5 mg orally once daily for 7 days

CASE SCENARIO 78

A 45-year-old female patient was diagnosed with hypertension 5 year back. She was maintained on Tab Amlodipine 10 mg once daily. She came to her physician with complaints of swelling over legs and fatigue for 20 days. Her BP was 160/90 mm Hg. ECG was normal. Blood urea and serum creatinine were also normal. Write a prescription for this patient incorporating all the elements.

Dr XY Jain
MBBS, MD (General Medicine)
Registration no. MPMC 223344
25, Park Street, Gwalior MP
Tel. no. 111222 Email: -------@-----.com

Date: 00.00.0000

Patient's name: Ms X
Age & Sex: 45 years, Female
Address: .... Weight: ....

Diagnosis: Moderate Hypertension

R_x
Tab Telmisartan 40 mg orally once daily for 7 days
Tab Metoprolol 50 mg orally once daily for 7 days
Salt restricted diet
Regular brisk walking for at least 30 min per day
Review after 7 days

XY Jain
Stamp

Alternative Agents

Tab Lisinopril 10 mg orally once daily. Tab Chlorthalidone 12.5 mg orally once daily for 7 days

CASE SCENARIO 79

A 42-year-old woman consults her family doctor as she has planned a trip by ship. As she has developed motion sickness on previous trips, she requests her doctor to give her a transdermal patch that is effective for this problem about which she has heard from a friend. Write a prescription for this patient incorporating all the elements.

Dr XY Jain
MBBS, MD (General Medicine)
Registration no. MPMC 223344
25, Park Street, Gwalior MP
Tel. no. 111222 Email: -------@-----.com

Date: 00.00.0000

Patient's name: Ms X
Age & Sex: 42 years, Female
Address: .... Weight: ....

Diagnosis: Motion Sickness

R_x

Hyoscine Hydrobromide skin patch 1.5 mg transdermal patch to be applied locally behind the ear 4 hr before start of journey

Repeat the same after 72 hr if required

XY Jain
Stamp

Alternative Agents

Tab Hyoscine Hydrobromide 300 mcg orally once 30 min before start of journey. Repeat after 2 hr if required OR

Tab Dimenhydrinate 50 mg orally single dose 1 hr before start of journey OR

Tab Meclizine 25 mg orally single dose 1 hr before start of journey OR

Tab Cinnarizine 25 mg orally single dose 2 hrs before start of journey

CASE SCENARIO 80

A 55-year-old male presented to skin outpatient department with multiple red raised asymptomatic lesions over the body for two months. Clinical examination revealed multiple asymptomatic erythematous plaques and well-circumscribed nodules of size 1.5–2 cm, over the forehead, nose, cheeks and both upper limbs. Bilateral ulnar nerves were thickened, and nontender. The skin lesions showed loss of hot, cold and touch sensations. Lepromin skin test was negative. Biopsy from the lesion showed the presence of diffuse infiltrate of macrophages and foamy cells, with few lymphocytes and plasma cells suggestive of tuberculoid leprosy. Slit skin smear showed acid-fast bacilli (*M. leprae*). Write a prescription for this patient incorporating all the elements.

Dr XY Jain
MBBS, MD (General Medicine)
Registration no. MPMC 223344
25, Park Street, Gwalior MP
Tel. no. 111222 Email: -------@-----.com

Date: 00.00.0000

Patient's name: Mr X
Age & Sex: 55 years, Male
Address: .... Weight: ....

Diagnosis: Multibacillary Leprosy

R_x
Tab Rifampin 600 mg orally once a month on empty stomach
Tab Clofazimine 50 mg orally once daily for 1 month and 300 mg orally once a month
Tab Dapsone 100 mg orally once daily for 1 month
To come for regular follow up every month
The colour of body secretions turns red with intake of Rifampicin
To report immediately in case of skin reaction
Refills: 11

XY Jain
Stamp

Alternative Agents to Clofazimine

Tab Ethionamide 250 mg plus Tab INH 300 mg orally once daily OR
Tab Minocycline 100 mg orally once daily OR
Tab Ofloxacin 400 mg orally once daily

CASE SCENARIO 81

A 65-year-old woman presented to her physician with complaints of bilateral drooping eyelids and double vision for the past two weeks. The woman also complained of slurring of speech on continued talking, difficulty in swallowing and intermittent weakness in her arms. Her symptoms were worse in the evenings and improved with rest and sleep. She had notable ptosis of both eyelids. Electromyographic testing revealed a decrementing muscle response to repetitive 2- or 3-Hz stimulation of motor nerves. An IV dose of 2 mg of edrophonium improved her symptoms. Write a prescription for this patient incorporating all the elements.

Dr XY Jain
MBBS, MD (General Medicine)
Registration no. MPMC 223344
25, Park Street, Gwalior MP
Tel. no. 111222 Email: -------@-----.com

Date: 00.00.0000

Patient's name: Ms X
Age & Sex: 65 years, Female
Address: .... Weight: ....

Diagnosis: Myasthenia Gravis

R_X
Tab Pyridostigmine 60 mg orally 8 hrly for 15 days
Tab Prednisolone 10 mg orally once a day for 15 days
Review after 15 days

XY Jain
Stamp

Alternative Agents to Pyridostigmine

Tab Neostigmine 15 mg orally 8 hrly for 15 days OR
Tab Ambenonium 5 mg orally 6 hrly for 15 days

Note: Adjuvants as per requirement
Tab Azathioprine 100 mg orally once daily for 15 days OR
Tab Cyclosporine 250 mg orally 12 hrly for 15 days

CASE SCENARIO 82

A 35-year-old male from an urban slum area develops subcutaneous nodules across his head and arms, after which he begins to experience frequent headaches with occasional nausea and vomiting. He had two sudden attacks of seizures 3 days apart. His seizures were generalized and tonic clonic, lasted for about 3 minutes each time and associated with tongue bite and micturition. He has no history of trauma. On questioning, he told that sometimes he used to take pork meat. On examination, the patient was alert and conscious. His vital signs were normal. Cardiovascular, respiratory and gastrointestinal systems were within normal limit. Investigations revealed normal haematological parameters. A computed tomography (CT) scan revealed one viable cystic lesion and one calcified lesion in the right frontal lobe of the brain. Blood ELISA test was positive for IgG antibodies for cysticercosis. Write a prescription for this patient incorporating all the elements.

Dr XY Jain
MBBS, MD (General Medicine)
Registration no. MPMC 223344
25, Park Street, Gwalior MP
Tel. no. 111222 Email: -------@-----.com

Date: 00.00.0000

Patient's name: Mr X
Age & Sex: 35 years, Male
Address: .... Weight: ....

Diagnosis: Neurocysticercosis

R_x
Tab Albendazole 400 mg orally 12 hrly for 8 days
Tab Sodium Valproate 750 mg orally once daily for 14 days
Tab Prednisolone 40 mg orally once daily for 10 days then
20 mg orally once daily for 10 days then
10 mg orally once daily for 10 days
Start Prednisolone two days before Albendazole
Review after 14 days

XY Jain
Stamp

Alternative Agents to Albendazole

Tab Praziquantel 600 mg orally 8 hrly for 15 days

Alternative Agents to Prednisolone

Tab Dexamethasone 8 mg orally daily for 30 days

CASE SCENARIO 83

A 56-year-old male presented to respiratory OPD with complaints of cough with sputum, pleuritic chest pain, and generalized weakness, loss of weight and loss of appetite for 2 months. On examination, blood pressure was 124/82 mm Hg, respiratory rate was 28 per min, temperature was 101°F. Respiratory findings revealed bilateral normal vesicular breath sounds with bilateral crepitations scattered throughout both the lung fields. X-ray chest showed bilateral pleural effusion with underlying consolidation. Sputum and bronchoalveolar lavage (BAL) sample were positive for weak, acid-fast, filamentous bacilli suggestive of Nocardia. Write a prescription for this patient incorporating all the elements.

Dr XY Jain
MBBS, MD (General Medicine)
Registration no. MPMC 223344
25, Park Street, Gwalior MP
Tel. no. 111222 Email: -------@-----.com

Date: 00.00.0000

Patient's name: Mr X
Age & Sex: 56 years, Male
Address: .... Weight: ....

Diagnosis: Nocardiosis

R_x
Tab Trimethoprim/Sulfamethoxazole 160/800 mg orally 12 hrly for 1 month
Tab Paracetamol 500 mg 6–8 hrly as required for fever
Review after 1 month
Refills: 5

XY Jain
Stamp

Alternative Agents

Inj Imipenem 500 mg IV 6 hrly till required then switch to
Tab Trimethoprim/Sulfamethoxazole 160/800 mg orally 12 hrly for 6 months OR
Inj Amikacin 250 mg IV 12 hrly till required then switch to
Tab Trimethoprim/Sulfamethoxazole 160/800 mg orally 12 hrly for 6 months OR
Tab Minocycline 100 mg orally 12 hrly for 6 months

CASE SCENARIO 84

A 35-year-old married female was referred to a clinical psychologist by her family physician. She reported about her compulsively repeating some acts in her daily life as an obsession. She supposed that her act of repeating some actions was a result of some specific persistent thoughts. She was obsessed with dirt and cleanliness. She used to wash her hands many times a day as indicated by her bleeding knuckles. She became so obsessed with cleanliness that she wanted to wash anything she touched. Her physical examination and blood tests were normal. Write a prescription for this patient incorporating all the elements.

Dr XY Jain
MBBS, MD (Psychiatry)
Registration no. MPMC 223344
25, Park Street, Gwalior MP
Tel. no. 111222 Email: -------@-----.com

Date: 00.00.0000

Patient's name: Ms X
Age & Sex: 35 years, Female
Address: .... Weight: ....

Diagnosis: Obsessive Compulsive Disorder

R_x
Tab Fluoxetine 20 mg orally once daily for 15 days
Review after 15 days

XY Jain
Stamp

Alternative Agents

Tab Clomipramine 20 mg orally once daily for 15 days OR
Tab Fluvoxamine 50 mg orally once daily for 15 days OR
Tab Sertraline 50 mg orally once daily for 15 days OR
Tab Paroxetin 20 mg orally once daily for 15 days OR
Tab Escitalopram 10 mg orally once daily for 15 days

CASE SCENARIO 85

A 55-year-old man consults a dermatologist for a persistent problem with his toenails for four months. All of his nails on both feet have brownish-black discoloration. On examination, the nails appear lustreless, brittle, hard, hypertrophic and the substance of the nail is friable. The patient has tried some topical ointments without any success. Write a prescription for this patient incorporating all the elements.

Dr XY Jain
MBBS, MD (Skin & VD)
Registration no. MPMC 223344
25, Park Street, Gwalior MP
Tel. no. 111222 Email: -------@-----.com

Date: 00.00.0000

Patient's name: Mr X
Age & Sex: 55 years, Male
Address: .... Weight: ....

Diagnosis: Onychomycosis

R_X
Tab Terbinafine 250 mg orally once daily for 1 month
Review after 1 month
Refills: 2

XY Jain
Stamp

Alternative Agents

Tab Fluconazole 150 mg orally once weekly for 6 months OR
Tab Itraconazole 200 mg orally once daily for 3 months

CASE SCENARIO 86

A 60-year-old man is found to have increased intraocular pressure in the right eye on eye examination. The visual acuity is normal in both eyes. Eye examination under mydriasis reveals increased cup-to-disc ratio in the right eye with no evidence of optic nerve damage. Mild loss of peripheral vision is found on perimetry test. Write a prescription for this patient incorporating all the elements.

Dr XY Jain
MBBS, MS (Ophthalmology)
Registration no. MPMC 223344
25, Park Street, Gwalior MP
Tel. no. 111222 Email: -------@-----.com

Date: 00.00.0000

Patient's name: Mr X
Age & Sex: 60 years, Male
Address: .... Weight: ....

Diagnosis: Open Angle Glaucoma

R_x
Betaxolol eye drops 0.5% one drop apply locally 12 hrly for 7 days
Review after 7 days

XY Jain
Stamp

Alternative Agents

Timolol eye drops 0.5% one drop apply locally 12 hrly for 7 days OR

Latanoprost eye drops 0.005% one drop apply locally once daily at night for 7 days OR

Bimatoprost eye drops 0.03% one drop apply locally once daily at night for 7 days OR

Travoprost eye drops 0.004% one drop apply locally once daily at night for 7 days

CASE SCENARIO 87

A 25-year-old man is brought to the emergency department. He is deeply unconscious, cyanosed and the pupils are markedly constricted. On examination, his heart rate is 62 beats per minute and respiratory rate is 7 per minute and shallow. On examination, his pupils are pinpoint and not reactive to light. There are multiple intravenous track marks on his arms bilaterally. On asking relatives informed that patient was dug addict but could not name the drug. The emergency physician diagnoses it as a case of a drug overdose. Patient was admitted in medicine ward. Write a prescription for this patient incorporating all the elements.

Dr XY Jain
MBBS, MD (General Medicine)
Registration no. MPMC 223344
25, Park Street, Gwalior MP
Tel. no. 111222 Email: -------@-----.com

Date: 00.00.0000

Patient's name: Mr X
Age & Sex: 25 years, Male
Address: .... Weight: ....

Diagnosis: Opioid Toxicity

R_X

Intermittent positive pressure respiration to establish airway

Gastric lavage by pot permanganate 1:5000 solution. Give 150 mL every 30 sec and aspirate till the colour of pot permanganate in aspirate remains pink

Dextrose 5% IV 5 mL/min

Inj Naloxone 1 mg IV stat and repeated every 5 min as needed to awaken the patient and maintain airway protective reflexes to a total dose of 10 mg

XY Jain
Stamp

CASE SCENARIO 88

A 30-year-old female complained of 3–4 vomiting in a day and more so in the morning. She gave a history of pregnancy for two and a half months. She also lost some weight. Physical examination revealed no pallor of conjunctiva and icterus. BP was 120/80 mm of Hg and pulse rate 80/min. Write a prescription for this patient incorporating all the elements.

Dr XY Jain
MBBS, MS (Obst & Gynae)
Registration no. MPMC 223344
25, Park Street, Gwalior MP
Tel. no. 111222 Email: -------@-----.com

Date: 00.00.0000

Patient's name: Ms X
Age & Sex: 30 years, Female
Address: .... Weight: ....

Diagnosis: Morning Sickness

R_x
Tab Doxylamine succinate 10 mg orally once at night for 7 days
Eat something before getting out of bed in the morning
Smaller frequent meals
Review after 7 days

XY Jain
Stamp

CASE SCENARIO 89

A 32-year-old male patient reported to the outpatient dental clinic with complaints of pain and burning sensation in the mouth for 15 days which were sudden in onset, moderate in intensity, constant in nature and aggravated while having hot and spicy food. There was no medical and drug history revealed. On intraoral examination, the lesion appeared creamy-white in colour without elevation seen on the hard and soft palate, measured approximately 5 × 3 cm in size. On palpation, the lesion was non-tender and scrapable. Brush biopsy of the lesion revealed intraepithelial pseudomycelia of *Candida albicans*. Patient was not immunocompromised. Write a prescription for this patient incorporating all the elements.

Dr XY Jain
MBBS, MD (General Medicine)
Registration no. MPMC 223344
25, Park Street, Gwalior MP
Tel. no. 111222 Email: -------@-----.com

Date: 00.00.0000

Patient's name: Mr X
Age & Sex: 32 years, Male
Address: .... Weight: ....

Diagnosis: Oral Candidiasis

R_x
Tab Fluconazole 100 mg orally once daily for 7 days
Clotrimazole lotion 1% apply locally with a cotton bud 8 hrly for 7 days

XY Jain
Stamp

Alternative to Fluconazole

Tab Ketoconazole 200 mg orally once daily for 7 days OR
Tab Itraconazole 200 mg orally once daily for 7 days

Alternative to Clotrmazole Lotion

Miconazole gel 2.5 ml apply locally 6 hourly for 7 days OR
Nystatin mouth rinses 4–6 ml (400,000 to 600,000 Units) held in the mouth before swallowing 8 hrly for 7 days

CASE SCENARIO 90

A 35-year-old male presented to the emergency department with a history of ingestion of unknown quantity of a household insecticide which was followed by multiple episodes of vomiting and breathing difficulty. There was no history of seizures. On examination, he was conscious and restless with both pupils pinpoint. His blood pressure 96/62 mm Hg, pulse 58/minute, respiratory rate 30/minute with excessive oral secretions. Deep tendon reflexes were sluggish. Patient was admitted in medicine ward. Write treatment for this patient.

Dr XY Jain
MBBS, MD (General Medicine)
Registration no. MPMC 223344
25, Park Street, Gwalior MP
Tel. no. 111222 Email: -------@-----.com

Date: 00.00.0000

Patient's name: Mr X
Age & Sex: 35 years, Male
Address: .... Weight: ....

Diagnosis: Organophosphate Poisoning

Rx

Inj Atropine 2 mg IV stat and then repeat every 5 minutes until dryness of mouth occurs max dose 200 mg

Inj Pralidoxime 1 g in 100 mL normal saline IV over 30 min

Repeat after 1 hr in the same dose, if required, up to max 12 g in 24 hr

Admit patient in aerated room. Check vitals at regular interval

XY Jain
Stamp

CASE SCENARIO 91

A 60-year-old female, weighing 65 kg, presents with pain in the right knee which started 6 months back. The pain was insidious in onset. She states that the pain is aggravated by walking and climbing stairs and is relieved by rest. The pain is associated with a limited range of movements in the right knee. She tells that similar complaint developed in the left knee one month back but it was mild. There is no history of trauma. X-ray of the right knee reveals joint space narrowing, subchondral sclerosis and osteophytes. Write a prescription for this patient incorporating all the elements.

Dr XY Jain
MBBS, MS (Orthopaedics)
Registration no. MPMC 223344
25, Park Street, Gwalior MP
Tel. no. 111222 Email: -------@-----.com

Date: 00.00.0000

Patient's name: Ms X
Age & Sex: 60 years, Female
Address: .... Weight: ....

Diagnosis: Osteoarthritis

Rx
Tab Paracetamol 500 mg orally 6 hrly for 7 days
Review after 7 days
Avoid squatting posture

XY Jain
Stamp

Other First Line Agents

Tab Naproxen 500 mg orally 12 hrly for 7 days OR
Tab Diclofenac 75 mg orally 12 hrly for 7 days OR
Tab Ibuprofen 400 mg orally 6 hrly for 7 days OR
Cap Indomethacin 50 mg orally 12 hrly for 7 days

CASE SCENARIO 92

A 68-year-old female attends orthopaedic OPD with complaint of diffuse bone pain for the last 2 months. She states any weight-bearing activity causes her severe discomfort. She has a history of hypertension for which she is taking hydrochlorothiazide 25 mg orally daily for the last two year. Her bone mineral density T-score is –2.6 at the hip and –2.0 at the spine. Write a prescription for this patient incorporating all the elements.

Dr XY Jain
MBBS, MS (Orthopaedics)
Registration no. MPMC 223344
25, Park Street, Gwalior MP
Tel. no. 111222 Email: -------@-----.com

Date: 00.00.0000

Patient's name: Ms X
Age & Sex: 68 years, Female
Address: .... Weight: ....

Diagnosis: Osteoporosis

R_x
Tab Alendronate 5 mg orally once daily for one month
Take half an hr before first food or drink with full glass of water and remain in sitting posture at least for 30 min to avoid oesophagitis
Treatment will be continued based on response
Review after one month

XY Jain
Stamp

Alternative Agents

Tab Alendronate 70 mg orally once weekly for one month OR
Tab Ibandronate 150 mg orally once a month OR
Tab Risedronate 35 mg orally once weekly for one month OR
Tab Risedronate 150 mg orally once a month OR
Inj Zolendronate 5 mg IV slow infusion in 15 min once a year

CASE SCENARIO 93

A 62-year-old man noticed progressively worsening tremors in his hands as well as rigidity involving the right side and bradykinesia for the past 6 months. The tremors were noticed at rest and disappeared with activity. He walked slowly and also developed slowness in his daily activities. His gait is characterized by small shuffling steps and a loss of the normal automatic arm swing. A right-sided resting tremor of the pill-rolling type was observed, which decreased during finger-to-nose coordination testing. A cogwheel rigidity was elicited by passively bending both arms. Write a prescription for this patient incorporating all the elements.

Dr XY Jain
MBBS, MD (General Medicine)
Registration no. MPMC 223344
25, Park Street, Gwalior MP
Tel. no. 111222 Email: -------@-----.com

Date: 00.00.0000

Patient's name: Mr X
Age & Sex: 62 years, Male
Address: .... Weight: ....

Diagnosis: Parkinsonism

R_x

Tab Levodopa/Carbidopa (250/25 mg) orally 8 hrly for 15 days
Review after 15 days

XY Jain
Stamp

Alternative Agents

Tab Pramipexole 0.25–1 mg orally 8 hrly OR
Tab Ropinirole 2 mg orally 8 hrly OR
Tab Selegiline 5 mg orally 12 hrly OR
Tab Rasagiline 1 mg orally once daily OR
Tab Entacapone 200 mg orally 8 hrly with each Levodopa/Carbidopa dose OR
Tab Tolcapone 100 mg orally 8 hrly with each Levodopa/Carbidopa dose OR
Tab Trihexyphenidyl 2 mg orally 8 hrly

CASE SCENARIO 94

A 30-year-old man reported a large single, hypopigmented, well-defined anaesthetic lesion on his right thigh which had been present for six months. His vitals were normal. On local examination there was a well-defined, hypopigmented, macule of 5 cm with anhidrosis and a raised granular margin associated with decreased sensation of touch, temperature and pain. There was no other nerve involvement. Lepromin skin test was positive. Biopsy from the lesion showed the presence of numerous epithelioid granulomas in the superficial and deep dermis. Slit skin smear showed acid-fast bacilli (*M. leprae*).Write a prescription for this patient incorporating all the elements.

Dr XY Jain
MBBS, MD (Skin & VD)
Registration no. MPMC 223344
25, Park Street, Gwalior MP
Tel. no. 111222 Email: -------@-----.com

Date: 00.00.0000

Patient's name: Mr X
Age & Sex: 30 years, Male
Address: .... Weight: ....

Diagnosis: Paucibacillary Leprosy

R_x
Tab Rifampicin 600 mg orally once a month
Tab Dapsone 100 mg orally once daily for one month
To report immediately in case of skin reaction
The color of body secretions will turn red with intake of Rifampicin
Regular follow up every month
Refills: 5

XY Jain
Stamp

CASE SCENARIO 95

A mother of 10-year-old child came to the physician with complaints of presence of lice and itching over scalp of her child who is otherwise asymptomatic. Write a prescription for this patient incorporating all the elements.

Dr XY Jain
MBBS, MD (Skin & VD)
Registration no. MPMC 223344
25, Park Street, Gwalior MP
Tel. no. 111222 Email: -------@-----.com

Date: 00.00.0000

Patient's name: Ms X
Age & Sex: 10 years, Male
Address: .... Weight: ....

Diagnosis: Pediculosis

R_X

Permethrin 1% lotion apply on scalp, allow to remain for 10 minutes then wash with water

Repeat the same after 7–10 days if lice are detected again.

XY Jain
Stamp

CASE SCENARIO 96

A 74-year-old woman presented to her family physician complaining of epigastric pain for 15 days. The pain occurred daily, was well localized, dull, non-radiating and increased at night and between meals. The patient reported relief of pain with antacids. She had been suffering from osteoarthritis for 3 months and had been taking ibuprofen two to three times daily to relieve her pain. On examination, her vitals were normal. Abdominal examination showed normal bowel sounds and mild epigastric tenderness. Upper endoscopy revealed a 4 cm clean-based gastric ulcer, and a biopsy of the ulcer site identified *Helicobacter pylori*. Write a prescription for this patient incorporating all the elements.

Dr XY Jain
MBBS, MD (General Medicine)
Registration no. MPMC 223344
25, Park Street, Gwalior MP
Tel. no. 111222 Email: -------@-----.com

Date: 00.00.0000

Patient's name: Ms X
Age & Sex: 74 years, Female
Address: .... Weight: ....

Diagnosis: Peptic Ulcer (*Helicobacter pylori*)

R_x
Cap Omeprazole 40 mg orally 12 hrly for 14 days
Tab Clarithromycin 500 mg orally 12 hrly for 14 days
Cap Amoxycillin 1 g orally 12 hrly for 14 days

Followed by
Cap Omeprazole 40 mg once daily before breakfast for 6 weeks

XY Jain
Stamp

Alternative Agents to Omeprazole

Tab Rabeprazole 20 mg orally once daily before breakfast for 6 weeks OR
Cap Lansoprazole 30 mg orally once daily before breakfast for 6 weeks OR
Tab Pantoprazole, 40 mg orally once daily before breakfast for 6 weeks

Alternative Triple Therapy Regimen

Cap Omeprazole 40 mg orally 12 hrly for 14 days
Cap Amoxycillin 1 g orally 12 hrly for 14 days
Tab Metronidazole 400 mg orally 8 hrly for 14 days

CASE SCENARIO 97

A 35-year-old male presents with swollen gums, bleeding from gums, pain on eating something hard, difficulty in chewing food, pus discharge from gum on pressing and loosening of teeth. He also complains of bad breath (halitosis) and sensitivity to hot and cold intakes. There is slowly progressive destruction of periodontium, loss of periodontal attachment with presence of periodontal pocket. Write a prescription for this patient incorporating all the elements.

Dr XY Jain
MBBS, MD (General Medicine)
Registration no. MPMC 223344
25, Park Street, Gwalior MP
Tel. no. 111222 Email: -------@-----.com

Date: 00.00.0000

Patient's name: Mr X
Age & Sex: 35 years, Male
Address: .... Weight: ....

Diagnosis: Periodontitis

Rx
Cap Amoxicillin 250 mg orally 8 hrly for 7 days
Tab Metronidazole 400 mg orally 8 hrly for 7 days
Tab Ibuprofen 400 mg orally 8 hrly for 5 days
Chlorhexidine mouthwash 0.2% 12 hrly

XY Jain
Stamp

Alternative Agents to Amoxicillin

Cap Doxycycline 100 mg orally 12 hrly for 7 days OR
Tab Ciprofloxacin 500 mg orally 12 hrly for 7 days OR
Cap Tetracycline 250 mg orally 6 hrly for 7 days OR
Tab Azithromycin 500 mg once daily for 3 days

Alternative Agents to Metronidazole

Tab Tinidazole 300 mg orally 12 hrly for 7 days

CASE SCENARIO 98

A 46-year-old woman presents with a dry hacking, prolonged, paroxysmal cough for the last 2 weeks. She states that the coughing spells are difficult to stop, and her sleep is often interrupted by coughing. She also reported occasional wheezing and chest tightness. During physical examination, the patient has several episodes of numerous rapid coughs, each followed by an inspiratory effort that includes a high-pitched whoop. On physical examination, her temperature 99.4°F, heart rate 94 beats per minute, blood pressure 140/90 mm Hg and oxygen saturation 98%. On lung auscultation, chest sounds clear. Culture of nasopharyngeal swab showed growth of *Bordetella pertussis*. Write a prescription for this patient incorporating all the elements.

Dr XY Jain
MBBS, MD (General Medicine)
Registration no. MPMC 223344
25, Park Street, Gwalior MP
Tel. no. 111222 Email: -------@-----.com

Date: 00.00.0000

Patient's name: Ms X
Age & Sex: 46 years, Female
Address: .... Weight: ....

Diagnosis: Pertussis

Rx
Tab Azithromycin 500 mg orally on day 1 followed by:
Tab Azithromycin 250 mg orally once daily for 4 days

XY Jain
Stamp

Alternative Agents

Tab Erythromycin 500 mg orally 6 hrly for 7 days OR
Tab Clarithromycin 500 mg orally 12 hrly for 7 days OR
Tab Trimethoprim/Sulfamethoxazole 160/800 mg orally 12 hrly for 7 days

CASE SCENARIO 99

A 34-year-old female presented with complaints of sudden onset and worsening symptoms of fever, chills, fatigue, nausea, vomiting, myalgia, productive cough and dyspnoea. The symptoms began the day before her hospital visit and severely worsened overnight. On physical examination, her temperature was 102.5°F and respiratory rate was 24/minute. Chest X-rays showed bilateral infiltrates and consolidation consistent with pneumonia. Sputum culture showed the presence of *Yersinia pestis*. Write a prescription for this patient incorporating all the elements.

Dr XY Jain
MBBS, MD (General Medicine)
Registration no. MPMC 223344
25, Park Street, Gwalior MP
Tel. no. 111222 Email: -------@-----.com

Date: 00.00.0000

Patient's name: Ms X
Age & Sex: 34 years, Female
Address: .... Weight: ....

Diagnosis: Plague

R_x
Inj Streptomycin 1 g IM 12 hrly for 10 days
Tab Paracetamol 500 mg orally 6–8 hrly as required for fever

XY Jain
Stamp

Other First Line Agents

Inj Gentamicin 240 mg IV once daily for 10 days

Alternative Agents

Cap Doxycycline 100 mg orally 12 hrly for 10 days OR
Cap Tetracycline 500 mg orally 6 hrly for 10 days OR
Tab Ciprofloxacin 1 g orally 12 hrly for 10 days OR
Tab Levofloxacin 500 mg orally once daily for 10 days

CASE SCENARIO 100

A 60-year-old male presents to his family physician with complaints of fever, chills, malaise, dyspnea and productive cough for 5 days. The sputum is mucoid, purulent and blood-tinged. He also complains of pain in his right chest that is more intense during inspiration. On examination, his blood pressure 150/84 mm Hg, heart rate 114/minute, respiratory rate 24/minute and temperature 102.4°F. Auscultation of chest reveals bilateral bronchial breath sounds, rhonchi and inspiratory crackles. Gram stain of sputum specimen shows gram-positive diplococci. Sputum culture reveals growth of *Streptococcus pneumoniae*. Write a prescription for this patient incorporating all the elements.

Dr XY Jain
MBBS, MD (General Medicine)
Registration no. MPMC 223344
25, Park Street, Gwalior MP
Tel. no. 111222 Email: -------@-----.com

Date: 00.00.0000

Patient's name: Mr X
Age & Sex: 60 years, Male
Address: .... Weight: ....

Diagnosis: Pneumococcal Pneumonia

R_X
Cap Amoxicillin 500 mg orally 8 hrly for 7 days
Tab Bromhexine 8 mg orally 8 hrly
Tab Paracetamol 500 mg orally 6–8 hrly as required for fever

XY Jain
Stamp

Other First Line Agents

Tab Cefpodoxime 200 mg 12 hrly for 7 days

Alternative Agents if Allergy to Penicillin

Tab Azithromycin 500 mg orally once daily for 3 days OR
Tab Clarithromycin 500 mg orally 12 hrly for 7 days OR
Cap Doxycycline 100 mg orally 12 hrly for 7 days, OR
Tab Levofloxacin 750 mg orally once daily for 7 days OR
Tab Moxifloxacin 400 mg orally once daily for 7 days

CASE SCENARIO 101

A 45-year-old man presented to the clinic with complaints of fever, progressive dyspnoea, weight loss and dry cough for the last 2 months. He had been treated with broad-spectrum antibiotics for a presumed diagnosis of pneumonia without any relief and most recently had finished a course of amoxicillin for 7 days. He had noticed a significant decrease in appetite in the immediate past and has lost approximately 8–10 kg of weight. On examination, temperature was 102.5°F, respiratory rate was 38/min, pulse rate 110/min and blood pressure 128/84 mm Hg. Chest examination revealed wheezes, rhonchi and crepitations on both sides. Other systems were normal. *Pneumocystis jiroveci* was found in the sputum but he proved to be HIV negative. Write a prescription for this patient incorporating all the elements.

Dr XY Jain
MBBS, MD (General Medicine)
Registration no. MPMC 223344
25, Park Street, Gwalior MP
Tel. no. 111222 Email: -------@-----.com

Date: 00.00.0000

Patient's name: Mr X
Age & Sex: 45 years, Male
Address: .... Weight: ....

Diagnosis: *Pneumocystis jiroveci* Pneumonia

R_X
Tab Trimethoprim/Sulfamethoxazole 320/1600 mg orally 8 hrly for 21 days
Tab Prednisolone 40 mg orally 12 hrly for 5 days
40 mg orally once daily for 5 days
20 mg orally once daily for 11days

XY Jain
Stamp

Alternative Agents

Tab Clindamycin 600 mg orally 8 hrly for 21 days +
Tab Primaquine 30 mg orally once daily for 21 days OR
Inj Pentamidine 200 mg IV once daily for 21 days

CASE SCENARIO 102

A 29-year-old primigravida delivered healthy male baby and was given Inj Ergometrine 0.3 mg IM at the delivery of anterior shoulder. After 1 hr of delivery when patient was shifted in the ward she complained of excessive bleeding per vagina. Her blood pressure was 100/60 mm Hg. Pulse rate was 112/min. Write a prescription for this patient incorporating all the elements.

Dr XY Jain
MBBS, MS (Obstetrics & Gynaecology)
Registration no. MPMC 223344
25, Park Street, Gwalior MP
Tel. no. 111222 Email: -------@-----.com

Date: 00.00.0000

Patient's name: Ms X
Age & Sex: 29 years, Female
Address: .... Weight: ....

Diagnosis: Postpartum Haemorrhage

Rx
Inj Oxytocin 10 IU in 500 mL glucose at the rate of 10 mL/min till required
Inj Carboprost 250 mcg IM 2 hrly till required max 3 mg in 24 hr

XY Jain
Stamp

Alternative Agents

Inj Dinoprostone 0.25 mg IM 2 hrly till required OR
Tab Misoprostol 800 mcg sublingually OR
Inj Methylergonovine 0.2 mcg IM, repeat every 2 hrs (maximum 1 mg in 24 hrs)

CASE SCENARIO 103

A 32-year-old female presented to her family physician with a 5-day history of greenish, foul-smelling watery diarrhea, fever and abdominal pain. The diarrhea occurred 3 days after starting clindamycin therapy for a recent tooth extraction due to a dental abscess. Physical examination of the patient revealed heart rate 110/min, and blood pressure 130/86 mm Hg. Laboratory investigations showed leukocytosis. Stool specimen was positive for *C. difficile* toxin. Write a prescription for this patient incorporating all the elements.

Dr XY Jain
MBBS, MD (General Medicine)
Registration no. MPMC 223344
25, Park Street, Gwalior MP
Tel. no. 111222 Email: -------@-----.com

Date: 00.00.0000

Patient's name: Ms X
Age & Sex: 32 years, Female
Address: .... Weight: ....

Diagnosis: Pseudomembranous Colitis

R_x
Tab Fidaxomicin 200 mg orally 12 hrly for 10 days

XY Jain
Stamp

Alternative Agents

Cap Vancomycin 125 mg orally 6 hrly for 10 days OR
Tab Metronidazole 500 mg orally 8 hrly for 10 days

CASE SCENARIO 104

A 26-year-old male, weighing 55 kg, presented with one month history of cough with expectoration, fever, night sweats, chills, loss of appetite, retrosternal chest pain, dyspnea on exertion and weight loss. On physical examination, the patient appeared chronically ill and malnourished. On chest examination, a few post-tussive rales were noted at right apex posteriorly. X-ray chest revealed a patchy area of consolidation with a well-defined cavitary lesion in the right upper lobe. Sputum smear was positive for acid-fast bacilli. Write a prescription for this patient incorporating all the elements.

Dr XY Jain
MBBS, MD (General Medicine)
Registration no. MPMC 223344
25, Park Street, Gwalior MP
Tel. no. 111222 Email: -------@-----.com

Date: 00.00.0000

Patient's name: Mr X
Age & Sex: 26 years, Male
Weight: 55 kg
Address: ....

Diagnosis: Pulmonary Tuberculosis

R_x
Tab Isoniazid 300 mg orally once daily for 1 month
Cap Rifampicin 600 mg orally once daily on empty stomach for 1 month
Tab Pyrazinamide 750 mg orally 12 hrly daily for 1 month
Tab Ethambutol 1000 mg orally once daily for 1 month
Tab Pyridoxine 10 mg orally once daily for 1 month
Follow up after one month
Ophthalmic examination before starting Ethambutol therapy
Rifampicin makes colour of urine red
Refills: 1

XY Jain
Stamp

Note: Intensive phase: Treatment for 2 months.

To undergo sputum examination after 2 months and continue INH and Rifampicin for another 4 months as continuation phase.

CASE SCENARIO 105

A 60-year-old woman presents to an orthopedician with complaints of generalized muscle and joint pain for the past 1 year. She also has morning stiffness of joints that lasts more than 1 h every morning. She states that her joints of both hands are swollen and painful and that she has been taking ibuprofen and paracetamol to control her pain but in spite of that she has to restrict her physical activities due to pain. Her vital signs are normal. Physical examination reveals bilateral symmetrical swelling, tenderness, and warmth of the metacarpophalangeal and proximal interphalangeal joints of both hands and the metatarsophalangeal joints of the feet. Blood haematology shows raised erythrocyte sedimentation rate and rheumatoid factor. X-ray of hands and feet show narrowing of joint spaces and marginal erosion of the articular surfaces. Write a prescription for this patient incorporating all the elements.

Dr XY Jain
MBBS, MD (General Medicine)
Registration no. MPMC 223344
25, Park Street, Gwalior MP
Tel. no. 111222 Email: -------@-----.com

Date: 00.00.0000

Patient's name: Ms X
Age & Sex: 60 years, Female
Address: .... Weight: ....

Diagnosis: Rheumatoid Arthritis

Rx
Tab Ibuprofen 400 mg orally 8 hrly for 7 days
Tab Prednisolone 7.5 mg orally once daily for 7 days
Tab Methotrexate 10 mg orally once weekly for 7 days
Tab Folic Acid 1 mg orally once daily for 7 days except on the day of Methotrexate.
Review after 7 days for dose escalation

XY Jain
Stamp

Alternative Agent to Ibuprofen:

Tab Naproxen 500 mg orally 12 hrly

CASE SCENARIO 106

A 36-year-old man presented to the dermatology clinic with rashes of one-month duration that were extremely itchy, particularly at night. Physical examination revealed numerous small erythematous vesicles, pustules and wavy thread-like grey burrows measuring 1 to 10 mm in diameter distributed primarily around the wrists, ankles, umbilicus and interdigital spaces of the hands and feet. Dermoscopic examination of the burrows revealed distinctive brown-coloured triangular structures that were removed with a fine scalpel. Microscopic examination of the tissue revealed moving mites, eggs, and faecal pellets. Write a prescription for this patient incorporating all the elements.

Dr XY Jain
MBBS, MD (Skin & VD)
Registration no. MPMC 223344
25, Park Street, Gwalior MP
Tel. no. 111222 Email: -------@-----.com

Date: 00.00.0000

Patient's name: Mr X

Age & Sex: 36 years, Male

Address: .... Weight: ....

Diagnosis: Scabies

R_X

Tab Ivermectin 12 mg orally as a single dose to be repeated after 2 weeks.

Permethrin 5% cream apply once all over the body from the neck down up to toes after bathing then wash off after 8–12 hr

Repeat after 1 week

Apply to all members of the family

Disinfect the clothes and bed sheets by boiling or ironing

XY Jain
Stamp

Alternative Agents to Permethrin

Gamma benzene hexachloride 1% lotion apply below neck on entire body surface overnight to be washed off next morning after a thorough scrub bath.

CASE SCENARIO 107

A 28-year-old male was referred by his family physician to psychiatric unit of a tertiary care hospital, with complaints of hearing voices for the past 6 months, restlessness, irritability and loss of appetite. The patient experienced auditory hallucinations. He complained of hearing voices of people talking about him and engaged in third person conversations involving both a man and a woman. The patient stated that he felt unsafe and thought that people wanted to harm him. On examination, he looks tired, depressed and avoided eye contact. Physical examination showed a thin, dishevelled-looking man with very poor hygiene, who appeared much older than his stated age, with normal vitals. Write a prescription for this patient incorporating all the elements.

Dr XY Jain
MBBS, MD (Psychiatry)
Registration no. MPMC 223344
25, Park Street, Gwalior MP
Tel. no. 111222 Email: -------@-----.com

Date: 00.00.0000

Patient's name: Mr X
Age & Sex: 28 years, Male
Address: .... Weight: ....

Diagnosis: Schizophrenia

Rx
Tab Olanzapine 20 mg orally once daily for 15 days
Review after 15 days

XY Jain
Stamp

Alternative Agents

Tab Aripriprazole 10 mg orally once daily for 15 days OR
Tab Risperidone 2 mg orally once daily for 15 days OR
Tab Quetiapine 50 mg orally 12 hrly for 15 days OR
Tab Haloperidol 5 mg orally 12 hrly for 15 days

CASE SCENARIO 108

A 54-year-old male patient presented to the emergency department with a history of cobra bite on the right foot. The bite had occurred about 20 minutes earlier. On admission he had vomiting and difficulty in breathing. He was fully conscious and there was no ptosis or double vision. His blood pressure was 142/94 mm Hg, pulse rate was 106/min; respiratory rate was 20/min and SpO_2 was 95%. Local examination of the patient's right foot showed oedema, redness, hotness, swelling, tenderness and two puncture marks about half an inch apart on the dorsum of his right foot. Patient was admitted in casualty ward. Write a prescription for this patient incorporating all the elements.

Dr XY Jain
MBBS, MD (General Medicine)
Registration no. MPMC 223344
25, Park Street, Gwalior MP
Tel. no. 111222 Email: -------@-----.com

Date: 00.00.0000

Patient's name: Mr X
Age & Sex: 54 years, Male
Address: .... Weight: ....

Diagnosis: Snakebite

R_X

Anti-snake venom (ASV) 10 vials (100 mL) in 250 ml of normal saline IV start with 10–15 drops/min for 15 min and watch for reaction. Continue ASV drip if no signs of reaction and to be completed in 1 hr followed by second dose after 1 hr if there is no improvement

Inj Atropine 0.6 mg IV stat and then every 30 min max 5 dose

Inj Neostigmine 2 mg IV every 30 min max 5 dose

Monitor vital signs at 5 min interval.

XY Jain
Stamp

CASE SCENARIO 109

A 28-year-old woman was brought to the emergency department in an unconscious state following frequent generalized tonic clonic seizures of 2 hr duration. She gave a history of headache and high-grade fever for two days prior to the onset of seizures. There was no history of seizures or major neurological illnesses in the past. Examination revealed that she was febrile and comatose. Her blood pressure and respiration were normal and there was no neck stiffness. Haematological investigations were normal. Patient was admitted in neurology ward. Write a prescription for this patient incorporating all the elements.

Dr XY Jain
MBBS, MD (General Medicine)
Registration no. MPMC 223344
25, Park Street, Gwalior MP
Tel. no. 111222 Email: -------@-----.com

Date: 00.00.0000

Patient's name: Ms X
Age & Sex: 28 years, Female
Address: .... Weight: ....

Diagnosis: Status Epilepticus

R_X
Inj Lorazepam 4 mg IV in 2 min repeat after 10 min if required (max 3 doses)
Review every 10 min till control of seizures

XY Jain
Stamp

Alternative Agents

Inj Diazepam 10 mg IV slowly (given over 2–5 min) OR
Inj Midazolam 10 mg IM repeat after 10 min if required

Note: If seizures uncontrolled with above treatment Inj Fosphenytoin (20 mg/kg) IV at a rate of 50 mg/min.

If still seizures continue Inj Phenobarbital 10–20 mg/kg IV slowly (50 mg/min).

CASE SCENARIO 110

A 22-year-old unmarried female patient consults her gynaecologist with a complaint of delayed periods by 2–3 months for two years. On examination her height is 5′.3″ and weight is 80 kg and she has facial hair growth. Her T3, T4 and TSH levels are normal. Her USG reveals ovarian cysts of more than 14 mm in size (normal 10 mm). The blood test revealed elevated LH and normal FSH levels. Write a prescription for this patient incorporating all the elements.

Dr XY Jain
MBBS, MS (Obst & Gynae)
Registration no. MPMC 223344
25, Park Street, Gwalior MP
Tel. no. 111222 Email: -------@-----.com

Date: 00.00.0000

Patient's name: Ms X
Age & Sex: 22 years, Female
Address: .... Weight: ....

Diagnosis: Polycystic Ovarian Disease

R_x
Tab Metformin 500 mg orally once a day for 5 days
Tab Norethisterone 5 mg orally 12 hourly for 5 days
Weight reduction exercise OR regular brisk walking for half an hour daily
Follow up or review when the period starts

XY Jain
Stamp

CASE SCENARIO 111

A 28-year-old male patient presented to outpatient clinic with dark, flat-to-raised rashes on his lower abdomen and arms for 5 days. The patient also stated that he had a small, painless sore on the left side of his penis that appeared 3 weeks earlier. It then became an open sore over the next several days. On examination, he had a painless superficial ulcer on penis with a clean base and firm, indurated margins with associated painless enlarged inguinal lymph nodes, which were rubbery, discrete, and nontender. Serological screening established positive VDRL test. Write a prescription for this patient incorporating all the elements.

Dr XY Jain
MBBS, MD (General Medicine)
Registration no. MPMC 223344
25, Park Street, Gwalior MP
Tel. no. 111222 Email: -------@-----.com

Date: 00.00.0000

Patient's name: Mr X
Age & Sex: 28 years, Male
Address: .... Weight: ....

Diagnosis: Syphilis

R_X
Inj Benzathine Penicillin G 2.4 Million Units deep IM once weekly for 3 weeks
Give first injection after sensitivity test (AST)

XY Jain
Stamp

Alternative Agents

Inj Ceftriaxone 1 g IM once daily for 10 days OR
Cap Doxycycline 100 mg orally 12 hrly for 14 days OR
Cap Tetracycline 500 mg orally 6 hrly for 14 days

CASE SCENARIO 112

A 28-year-old male presented to his family physician after observing numerous intestinal tapeworms in feces. He complained of perianal itching, diffuse cramp-like abdominal pain and occasional diarrhea for two weeks. There was no fever. The patient referred to habitual intake of all kinds of raw meats and fish. The examination revealed mild pain on deep palpation of the right iliac fossa. Haematological test revealed mild eosinophilia. Microbiological examination of stool detected proglottids of taenia solium. Write a prescription for this patient incorporating all the elements.

Dr XY Jain
MBBS, MD (General Medicine)
Registration no. MPMC 223344
25, Park Street, Gwalior MP
Tel. no. 111222 Email: -------@-----.com

Date: 00.00.0000

Patient's name: Mr X
Age & Sex: 28 years, Male
Address: .... Weight: ....

Diagnosis: Taenia Solium Infestation

R_x
Tab Praziquantel 500 mg orally single dose

XY Jain
Stamp

Alternative Agents

Tab Niclosamide 500 mg 2 tabs orally with one glass of water on empty stomach then 2 tab after one h followed by

Tab Docusate 100 mg orally after 2 hr.

CASE SCENARIO 113

A 45-year-old female patient who was a known case of hyperthyroidism was treated with carbimazole. Patient stopped taking carbimazole herself one month back as she was feeling normal. She was brought to casualty department by her husband with complains of chest pain, palpitation, shortness of breath, tremor, nervousness, increased sweating, disorientation, fever and loose motions. On examination, her pulse rate was 112/minute with high pulse pressure. Patient was admitted in medicine ward. Write a prescription for this patient incorporating all the elements.

Dr XY Jain
MBBS, MD (General Medicine)
Registration no. MPMC 223344
25, Park Street, Gwalior MP
Tel. no. 111222 Email: -------@-----.com

Date: 00.00.0000

Patient's name: Ms X
Age & Sex: 45 years, Female
Address: .... Weight: ....

Diagnosis: Thyrotoxic Crisis

R_x
Inj Propranolol 1 mg IV 4 hrly
Tab Propylthiouracil 250 mg orally 6 hrly
Inj Hydrocortisone 100 mg IV 8 hrly
Potassium Iodide Solution 10 drops orally 8 hrly (begin one hour after the first dose of propylthiouracil)

XY Jain
Stamp

Alternative to IV Propranolol

Tab Propranolol 40–80 mg orally 6 hrly OR
Tab Diltiazem 90 mg orally 8 hrly OR
Inj Diltiazem 10 mg/hr IV

Note: Plasmapheresis or peritoneal dialysis to remove protein bound hormone if above measures fail to control disease.

CASE SCENARIO 114

A 21-year-old male presents with superficial lesions on his trunk. On examination, the man is found to have five roughly circular skin lesions on his body. The lesions range from 2 to 8 cm in diameter and have red, raised borders and central clearing. The centres of some lesions are hypopigmented. They are quite itchy, but not painful. His general physical examination is normal. Write a prescription for this patient.

Dr XY Jain
MBBS, MD (Skin & VD)
Registration no. MPMC 223344
25, Park Street, Gwalior MP
Tel. no. 111222 Email: -------@-----.com

Date: 00.00.0000

Patient's name: Mr X
Age & Sex: 21 years, Male
Address: .... Weight: ....

Diagnosis: Tinea Corporis

R_x
Tab Terbinafine 250 mg orally once daily for 4 weeks
Miconazole 2% cream apply locally 12 hrly for 2 weeks

XY Jain
Stamp

Alternative to Terbinafine

Tab Ketoconazole 200 mg orally once daily for 2–4 weeks OR
Tab Itraconazole 200 mg orally once daily for 2–4 weeks OR
Tab Fluconazole 200 mg orally once daily for 2–4 weeks

Alternative to Miconazole Cream

Clotrimazole 1% cream apply locally 12 hrly for 4 weeks
Terbinafine 1% cream apply locally once daily for 4 weeks

CASE SCENARIO 115

A 35-year-old man, weighing 68 kg, presented to his primary care physician with low grade fever, persistent headache, malaise, fatigue and painless swelling of the lymph nodes, of 6 months duration. Physical examination revealed enlarged, nontender, freely mobile bilateral cervical and inguinal lymph nodes measuring up to 3 cm. Ultrasonography of the abdomen showed a moderate splenomegaly. In serological testing Toxoplasma IgM with Toxoplasma IgG also being positive. Write a prescription for this patient incorporating all the elements.

Dr XY Jain
MBBS, MD (General Medicine)
Registration no. MPMC 223344
25, Park Street, Gwalior MP
Tel. no. 111222 Email: -------@-----.com

Date: 00.00.0000

Patient's name: Mr X
Age & Sex: 35 years, Male
Weight: 68 kg
Address: .... Weight: ....

Diagnosis: Toxoplasmosis

R_x
Tab Pyrimethamine 200 mg orally as first dose then 75 mg once daily for 6 weeks
Tab Sulfadiazine 1500 mg orally 6 hrly for 6 weeks
Tab Folinic Acid 10 mg orally once daily for 6 weeks
Tab Paracetamol 500 mg orally 6–8 hrly as required for fever

XY Jain
Stamp

Alternative Agents

Tab Clindamycin 600 mg orally 6 hrly for 6 weeks OR
Tab Trimethoprim/Sulfamethoxazole 160/800 mg orally 8 hrly for 6 weeks OR
Tab Azithromycin 1 g orally once daily for 6 weeks OR
Tab Clarithromycin 500 mg orally 12 hrly for 6 weeks

Toxoplasmosis during Pregnancy

Tab Spiramycin 1 g orally 8 hrly until delivery.

CASE SCENARIO 116

A 32-year-old female presents to her gynaecologist with a 5-day history of profuse yellow-green vaginal discharge with an unpleasant odour. She also has mild pelvic pain. On speculum examination, the discharge is green in colour and frothy in appearance with "strawberry" appearance of the cervix. Vaginal pH is 6.2. Microscopic examination of vaginal swab reveals *Trichomonas vaginalis*. Write a prescription for this patient incorporating all the elements.

Dr XY Jain
MBBS,M S (Obstetrics & Gynaecology)
Registration no. MPMC 223344
25, Park Street, Gwalior MP
Tel. no. 111222 Email: -------@-----.com

Date: 00.00.0000

Patient's name: Ms X
Age & Sex: 32 years, Female
Address: .... Weight: ....

Diagnosis: Trichomonal Vaginitis

Rx
Tab Metronidazole 400 mg orally 12 hrly for 7 days

XY Jain
Stamp

Alternative Agents

Tab Metronidazole 2 g orally single dose OR
Tab Tinidazole 2 g orally single dose OR
Tab Secnidazole 2 g orally single dose

Note: Because the *Trichomonas vaginalis* is a sexually transmitted infection treatment of both partners simultaneously is recommended.

CASE SCENARIO 117

A 42-year-old man is referred to the neurology clinic by his family physician with the chief complaint of severe intermittent episodes of lancinating pain on the right side of the face for the past one year. He states that it is a sharp stabbing pain radiating over his right cheek. The pain aggravates while chewing, brushing teeth, washing face, and even on touching. The pain is so intense that it disrupts his activities of daily living. He has tried paracetamol with no improvement. The intraoral and extraoral examinations are normal. Radiological investigation revealed no abnormalities. Write a prescription for this patient incorporating all the elements.

Dr XY Jain
MBBS, MD (General Medicine)
Registration no. MPMC 223344
25, Park Street, Gwalior MP
Tel. no. 111222 Email: -------@-----.com

Date: 00.00.0000

Patient's name: Mr X
Age & Sex: 42 years, Male
Address: .... Weight: ....

Trigeminal Neuralgia

Rx
Tab Carbamazepine 200 mg orally 12 hrly for 5 days

XY Jain
Stamp

Alternative Agents

Tab Oxcarbazepine 300 mg orally 12 hrly OR
Tab Topiramate 50 mg orall 12 hrly

CASE SCENARIO 118

A 54-year-old man presented with a 5-day history of sudden onset of a cutaneous lesion on his left knee, associated with fever, chills, headache, malaise, myalgia and inguinal lymphadenopathy. He gave a history of insect bite on his left knee, a few hr before initiation of the symptoms. On examination, his temperature was 103°F. Physical examination revealed the presence of a maculopapular rash on his left knee and a large, tender, fluctuant left inguinal lymph node with mildly enlarged adjacent lymph nodes. On serological test antibody titers to *F. tularensis* were 1:80. Blood culture was positive for *F. tularensis*. Write a prescription for this patient incorporating all the elements.

Dr XY Jain
MBBS, MD (General Medicine)
Registration no. MPMC 223344
25, Park Street, Gwalior MP
Tel. no. 111222 Email: -------@-----.com

Date: 00.00.0000

Patient's name: Mr X
Age & Sex: 54 years, Male
Address: .... Weight: ....

Diagnosis: Tularemia

R_x
Inj Streptomycin 1 g IM 12 hrly for 10 days

XY Jain
Stamp

Other First Line Agents

Inj Gentamicin 240 mg IV/IM once daily for 10 days

Alternative Agents

Cap Doxycycline 100 mg orally 12 hrly for 14 days OR
Cap Tetracycline 500 mg orally 6 hrly for 14 days

CASE SCENARIO 119

A 32-year-old male presented with complaints of a cyclic fever (102–103°F), chills, fatigue and a severe headache for the last seven days and non-bloody diarrhea associated with pain in abdomen and vomiting for three days. On physical examination, the patient appeared fatigued with dry mucous membranes. His temperature 102°F, blood pressure 96/68 mm Hg, heart rate 90/minute and respiratory rate 18/minute. Complete blood count revealed normocytic normochromic anemia (hemoglobin 9.3 g/dL) with leucopenia. His chest X-ray was normal. Blood culture was positive for *Salmonella typhi*. Three malaria smears were negative. Write a prescription for this patient incorporating all the elements.

Dr XY Jain
MBBS, MD (General Medicine)
Registration no. MPMC 223344
25, Park Street, Gwalior MP
Tel. no. 111222 Email: -------@-----.com

Date: 00.00.0000

Patient's name: Mr X
Age & Sex: 32 years, Male
Address: .... Weight: ....

Diagnosis: Typhoid Fever

R_X
Inj Ceftriaxone 2 g IV once daily for 14 days
Tab Paracetamol 500 mg 6–8 hrly as required for fever

XY Jain
Stamp

Alternative Agents

Tab Azithromycin 1 gm orally once daily for 5 days OR
Tab Trimethoprim/Sulfamethoxazole 160/800 mg orally 12 hrly for 14 days OR
Tab Ciprofloxacin 750 mg orally 12 hrly for 14 days OR
Tab Levofloxacin 500 mg orally once daily for 14 days OR
Cap Amoxicillin 1 g orally 8 hrly for 14 days OR
Tab Cefixime 400 mg orally 12 hrly for 14 days

CASE SCENARIO 120

A 35-year-old female, weighing 45 kg, presents with frequency, urgency and dysuria for the last 3 days. On examination, her temperature is 98.6°F, heart rate is 72/minute and blood pressure is 118/72. Microscopic examination of urine reveals presence of microorganisms. Write a prescription for this patient incorporating all the elements.

Dr XY Jain
MBBS, MD (General Medicine)
Registration no. MPMC 223344
25, Park Street, Gwalior MP
Tel. no. 111222 Email: -------@-----.com

Date: 00.00.0000

Patient's name: Ms X
Age & Sex: 35 years, Female
Address: .... Weight: ....

Diagnosis: Uncomplicated UTI

R_x
Tab Nitrofurantoin 100 mg orally 12 hrly for 7 days

XY Jain
Stamp

Alternative Agents

Tab Trimethoprim/Sulfamethoxazole (160/800 mg) orally 12 hrly for 7 days OR
Tab Ciprofloxacin 250 mg orally 12 hrly for 3 days OR
Tab Cephalaxin 500 mg orally twice daily for 5 days

CASE SCENARIO 121

A 65-year-old female presented to a urologist with complaints of urinary urgency, frequency, and nocturia for 6 months. She told that often she has sudden, intense urge to urinate, followed by an involuntary loss of urine. These incontinence issues greatly impacted her quality of life. She avoided social activities and long walks due to a fear of leaking. She has no history of dysuria or haematuria. Her abdominal and pelvic examinations were normal. Write a prescription for this patient incorporating all the elements.

Dr XY Jain
MBBS, MD (General Medicine)
Registration no. MPMC 223344
25, Park Street, Gwalior MP
Tel. no. 111222 Email: -------@-----.com

Date: 00.00.0000

Patient's name: Ms X
Age & Sex: 65 years, Female
Address: .... Weight: ....

Diagnosis: Urge Incontinence

R_x
Tab Tolterodine 1 mg orally 12 hrly for 15 days
Do daily pelvic floor exercises. Avoid lifting weight
Review after 15 days

XY Jain
Stamp

Alternative Agents

Tab Oxybutynin 2.5 mg orally 12 hrly for 15 days OR
Tab Darifenacin 7.5 mg orally once daily for 15 days OR
Tab Solifenacin 5 mg orally once daily for 15 days OR
Tab Mirabegron 25 mg orally once daily for 15 days

CASE SCENARIO 122

A 30-year-old woman is hospitalized in postoperative ward of a tertiary care hospital after caesarean section delivery of her first child. The child was born at term by caesarean section because of failure of labour to progress. The patient has been unable to void normally 4–6 hr after removal of catheter. Write a prescription for this patient incorporating all the elements.

Dr XY Jain
MBBS, MD (General Medicine)
Registration no. MPMC 223344
25, Park Street, Gwalior MP
Tel. no. 111222 Email: -------@-----.com

Date: 00.00.0000

Patient's name: Ms X
Age & Sex: 30 years, Female
Address: .... Weight: ....

Diagnosis: Urinary Retention (Postoperative Nonobstuctive)

R_x
Inj Neostigmine 0.5 mg IM stat

XY Jain
Stamp

Alternative Agents

Tab Bethanechol 25 mg orally 8 hrly on empty stomach until required

CASE SCENARIO 123

A 27-year-old full term pregnant woman was brought in labor room with pain in abdomen for three hours. On examination, obstetrician found her in first stage of labor. Ten hours after her admission pain in abdomen was not increased and cervix was 8 cm dilated. She had slight per vaginal discharge. Her uterine contractions were inadequate. Induction of labor was advised. Write a prescription for this woman.

Dr XY Jain
MBBS, MS (Obstetrics & Gynaecology)
Registration no. MPMC 223344
25, Park Street, Gwalior MP
Tel. no. 111222 Email: -------@-----.com

Date: 00.00.0000

Patient's name: Ms X
Age & Sex: 27 years, Female
Address: .... Weight: ....

Diagnosis: Uterine Inertia

Rx

Inj Oxytocin 5 International Units in 500 mL of 5% dextrose at the rate of 2–4 Milli International Units/min

Rate of infusion can be increased up to 20 Milli International Units /min with close monitoring of fetal heart and uterine contractions.

Not more than 5 International Units are to be administered in 24 hr

XY Jain
Stamp

Alternative Agents

Tab Dinoprostone 10 mg per vaginum (intravaginal) as a single dose. Remove the insert upon onset of active labor or 12 hours after insertion.

Direction: To remain in recumbent position during and up to 2 hr of insertion.

CASE SCENARIO 124

A 28-year-old female patient complains of itching and red spots over her body for 1 hour. The patient has a history of consumption of seafood one hour before. This is the first time the patient ate seafood. There is no history of any drug intake or any other skin disease in the past. Write a prescription for this patient incorporating all the elements.

Dr XY Jain
MBBS, MD (General Medicine)
Registration no. MPMC 223344
25, Park Street, Gwalior MP
Tel. no. 111222 Email: -------@-----.com

Date: 00.00.0000

Patient's name: Ms X
Age & Sex: 28 years, Female
Address: .... Weight: ....

Diagnosis: Urticaria

R_X
Tab Desloratadine 5 mg orally once daily for 5 days
Calamine lotion apply locally 12 hourly for 5 days
Avoid seafood.
Review after 5 days

XY Jain
Stamp

Alternative Agents

Tab Levocetrizine 5 mg orally once daily for five days

CASE SCENARIO 125

A 30-year-old female presented to her gynaecologist with a 5-day history of pain on urination, vaginal itching, and a thick, white creamy vaginal discharge. She denied having any allergies to medications or other medical conditions. Vaginal pH test revealed a pH of 4.2. Culture of vaginal swab showed growth of *Candida albicans*. Write a prescription for this patient incorporating all the elements.

Dr XY Jain
MBBS, MS (Obstetrics & Gynaecology)
Registration no. MPMC 223344
25, Park Street, Gwalior MP
Tel. no. 111222 Email: -------@-----.com

Date: 00.00.0000

Patient's name: Ms X
Age & Sex: 30 years, Female
Address: .... Weight: ....

Diagnosis: Vaginal Candidiasis

R_X
Tab Fluconazole 150 mg orally single dose after food
Clotrimazole vaginal pessary 100 mg apply intravaginally once daily for 6 days

XY Jain
Stamp

Alternative to Fluconazole

Tab Itraconazole 200 mg orally once daily for 3 days

Alternative to Clotrimazole

Miconazole vaginal pessary 100 mg intravaginally daily for 7 days OR
Terconazole 80 mg vaginal suppository intravaginally daily for 3 days OR
Tioconazole 6.5% ointment 5 g intravaginally in a single application

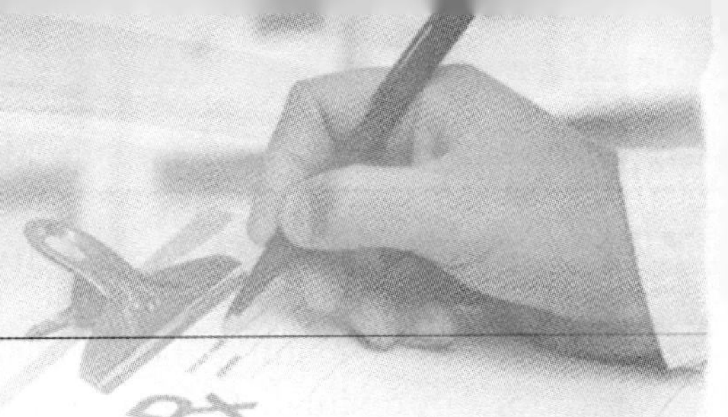

Chapter

3 Communication with Patients on Prescriptions

Need of Communication

Communication is the transfer of appropriate information from the prescriber to the patient either verbally or/and in writing. Prescription, though written carefully and correctly may be ineffective unless communicated properly to the patient and the pharmacists. Registered medical practitioners should have proper communication skill for successful prescribing and health care of society. Communication skill was not paid much attention in the old curriculum. It is an art that requires training so it has now been included in the revised curriculum. Training on communication at an early stage of education period to undergraduate medical students is essential to ensure

1. *Positive impact on patient–doctor relationship:* If the doctor gives attention to the patient's concern and addresses his expectation about his illness, a strong relationship between patient and doctor is built.
2. *Patient's satisfaction:* If the doctor listens patiently, gives sufficient time and then explains to him with empathy it results in better patient satisfaction.
3. *Compliance of the treatment:* When quality information is given to the patient then the patient will have a greater understanding of his problem and drugs given to him for treatment. This contributes to better adherence to treatment strategy. Elderly patients suffering from comorbidities and on multitherapy are at a higher risk of noncompliance.
4. *Prevention of drug prescription errors:* Positive interaction with patients encourages them to follow medical recommendations correctly, thereby preventing prescription errors.
5. *Confidence of the prescriber:* Improvement in patient-centered communication helps even better confidence in the doctor. It allows the physician to provide competent and economically prudent care within the accepted medical practice and to make treatment decisions which are in the best interest of the patient.
6. *Success of treatment:* Effective doctor–patient communication has shown a positive influence on health outcome.

Key points for effective communication skill: The amount of information given to patients will vary according to the nature of their condition. The important information provided to patients in the local language includes:

1. The name of the medicines and likely benefits from them.
2. The objective of the treatment.

3. Frequency and complexity of drug regimen and the total number of drugs, instructions for how to use inhalers or transdermal patches.
4. Advice to judge the benefit of the drug.
5. Approximate time expected to get improvement.
6. Duration of therapy and the grounds on which the decision is made to stop or change the treatment. Premature discontinuation of drugs may cause relapse especially in the case of treatment of infectious diseases.
7. Inform the most suitable timings to take drugs for better efficacy. *For example:* PPI should be taken on empty stomach and NSAIDs should be taken after meals.
8. Ask the patient about the previous allergy to any drugs.
9. Explain what adverse drug reactions (ADR) are possible with prescribed drugs. Orient them about likely risks, including serious and common side effects. It is likely that patient will not adhere to the drugs which cause confusion or altered mental status.
10. Tell them to report immediately, if ADR occurs.
11. Warn them to avoid taking any other drug which may interact with the present prescription, e.g. avoid alcohol when metronidazole is prescribed. Explain to them the reason to avoid.
12. Always share the next date of follow up consultation for the review of the treatment.
13. Instruct clearly how to taper drugs before stopping them especially when steroids are prescribed.
14. Ask them not to stop the drug abruptly when symptoms are relieved, assuming that there is no need to continue the drug, e.g. beta blockers in hypertension, sudden withdrawal may result in exacerbation of hypertension.
15. Instruct the patient about which food substances are to be avoided with drugs, e.g. tetracyclines should not be taken with milk.
16. Convey clearly when not to worry if some changes are noticed under medication, like urine colour may become dark in case of rifampicin, stool colour may be black in case of iron.
17. Communicate effectively on the method of use of devices for certain prescribed medications such as metered dose inhaler (MDI), spacer, nebulizer, insulin syringe, insulin self-administration, eye/ear/nose drops, application of the ointment, cream, transdermal patch and suppository, etc.
18. Patients should be informed about the proper storage of drugs. If the drugs are not stored properly they may lose efficacy, potency and safety.
19. Instruct to discard expired drugs because they may be less effective, ineffective or dangerous at times, e.g. Fancony syndrome is seen with the use of expired tetracycline.
20. Instruct them to keep drugs out of the reach of children.
21. Warn them not to take the drugs written on earlier prescription repeatedly without consulting the physician. It can be dangerous in the case of habit forming drugs like codeine in cough mixtures.
22. Do not change the dose strength of the drugs without consulting treating physician even when there is an improvement, e.g. in case of treatment of infection.
23. To take precautions, e.g. do not drive when taking first generation antihistamines.

24. Inform about the laboratory tests needed, e.g. prothrombin time with oral anticoagulants.
25. Avoid self-medication.
26. Communicate pregnant patients about the possible teratogenic effects of drugs to the fetus. Tell them to avoid such drugs in the first trimester of pregnancy, unless the benefit to the mother outweighs the risk to the fetus. Also mention that growth of the fetus or functional development may also be affected if drugs are used in the second and third trimester.
27. Involve the patients in decisions about their care and respect their autonomy. Discussing therapeutic options will encourage the patient to choose a suitable alternative and this will prevent them to abscond from getting treated.

Factors to be Considered while Prescribing Drugs Causing Dependence

Doctors should be extra careful in prescribing habit forming drugs to avoid their misuse. Only authorized practitioners can prescribe controlled substances; in such cases it might be necessary to indicate details of the authority on the prescription.

It is required for the prescriber to be aware of the characteristics of each drug, its accepted indications for use, and its general and specific risks while prescribing. It is a cause of concern that nonmedical uses of sedative-hypnotics and opioids are becoming a major threat to public health. People use them for pleasurable effects, relaxation and relief of distress. These substances work by altering the mind and there is a need to provide education and create awareness about the hazards of prescription drug's misuse. The doctor, dispenser, nurse and stockist all should take extra care and the following points should be considered:

1. Prescribers should inform the patient about these drugs potential for habit forming, as well as the dangers of long-term and excessive use. A single prescription for habit forming medicines can make a patients lifetime addict.
2. Fresh prescription order written on letterhead with authorized doctor's details, signature and date is mandatory before the sale of such drugs.

Table 3.1: The drugs causing dependence

S.no.	*Drug group*	*Name of drugs*
1	Benzodiazepines	Diazepam, Alprazolam, Lorazepam, Nitrazepam, Flurazepam, Midazolam, Clonazepam, Clobazam, Chlordiazepoxide
2	Barbiturates	Phenobarbitone, Pentobarbitone
3	Opioids	Morphine, Codeine, Dihydromorphinon Heroin, Pethidine, Pentazocine, Buprenorphine, Propoxyphene, Dextro-propoxyphene, Oxycodone/Tramadol
4	Club drugs	Methylenedioxymethamphetamine (MDMA), Flunitrazepam, Gamma-hydroxybutyrate (GHB)
5	Hallucinogens	Lysergic Acid Diethylamide (LSD), Mescaline, Psilocybin
6	Dissociative drugs	Ketamine, Phencyclidine
7	Stimulant drugs	Caffeine, Nicotine and Alcohol
8	Inhalants	Glue, nail varnish, petrol, paint solvents
9	Drugs use is illegal /illicit	Marijuana, Hashish, Cocaine, Amphetamine, Methamphetamine

3. The strength, frequency of administration and the total quantity of the control substance to be dispensed for the therapy should be stated clearly, further all quantities should be written in words as well as in figures to prevent any type of alterations. Other details such as patient's particulars and date of prescribing should also be filled in carefully to avoid alteration. Smaller quantities should be advised and the prescriber should also give direction to the dispenser: "Do not refill until instructed". It is advisable to give due justification for large quantities of a particular drug prescribed. The National Medical Commission is the authority to take action against the doctor who misuses his powers by prescribing large quantities of drugs causing dependence for other than judicious medical use. Pharmacists can refuse to dispense such prescriptions.
4. Overwriting in prescription is to be avoided. If needed for any reason, strike out the wrong word/quantity, write it afresh and countersign it.
5. Any change or corrections on the invoice should be avoided.
6. The medicine listed above in the table should not be advised verbally or given over the telephone through text messages (SMS) or E-mail to the patients. Pharmacists are not authorized to dispense these drugs against such orders and have the right of refusal to dispense.
7. Avoid prescribing opioids to patients with alcohol or substance use disorders. This substantially increases the risks of adverse effects, particularly cognitive impairment, sedation and respiratory depression.
8. Opioid medications should only be used for the treatment of the pain when non-opioid pain medications and therapies have failed or are likely to fail to provide adequate pain relief. After proper checking these drugs should be immediately shifted to a special cupboard, designated to stock only such drugs, and always kept under lock and key. The key should be with a responsible person.
9. *Instructions for the dispenser:* Dispenser needs to ensure that the prescription is genuine, complete and not having any manipulation or overwriting. Strictly, no verbal orders from a doctor/hospital should be entertained for such drugs.
    - To ensure that there is no misuse/repeat buying by the patient, the pharmacy man should put a "Dispensed" stamp without fail on the prescription.
    - The quantity sold against such orders must not be more than that ordered.
    - Dispensing/sale of such medicines cannot be done against the prescription of doctors of other systems of medicines or unauthorized persons/quacks, pharmacists or nurse.
    - The wholesaler must keep a hard copy of all the orders received from doctors/hospitals and retailers, and retain the same for at least two years.
    - The invoice should be complete with details of prescribing doctor and detailed information of the drug's batch number, price, etc. with the signature of the competent person.
    - One should always check and tally these drugs from time to time to ensure that there are no errors in handling.

Chapter

4

Common Prescription Errors

Causes of Prescription Errors

Prescribing is an important tool to control or treat diseases but can increase the sufferings of the patients on account of prescription errors. Studies have shown that approximately 50% of prescriptions have errors (WHO). Prescription errors may be associated with a number of reasons:

1. Lack of ability to diagnose the patient's problem.
2. Incomplete knowledge of existing or new drugs indicated for a particular disease as per local and national guidelines.
3. Lack of training to prescribe in special situations like comorbidity, pregnant patients, paediatric and geriatric patients.
4. Not following principles of prescribing.
5. Lack of effective communication skill with patients on prescription.
6. Prescribing decision is influenced by the salesmanship of drug manufacturers to push their products.

Incorrect prescribing practices can lead to unsafe, ineffective, unethical treatment, exacerbation or prolongation of disease, increased hospital stay and financial burden to the patients. Occasionally, it can result in fatal consequences.

The national medical commission has revised the medical curriculum and prepared a document outlining a framework of prescribing competency to impart good prescribing habits in medical students at second phase MBBS. It is not easy to prescribe safely and effectively amongst various drugs available unless a high level of knowledge, skill and training is ensured. It is important to learn correct prescribing skills to avoid prescribing errors.

Samples of Common Prescribing Errors

For problem-based learning, samples of prescriptions with different types of errors are being given. Students have to critically analyze and rewrite the correct prescriptions. Error reports and correction tips are provided at the end of the chapter for the readers to check their answers.

Sample 1

Date: 05.01.2021

Patient's name: Mr V
Age & Sex: 30 years, Male
Weight: 55 kg
Address: 24, Modern Colony, Gwalior

Diagnosis: Plague

R_x

Inj Streptomycin 1 g IM 12 hourly for 10 days
Tab Paracetamol 500 mg orally 6–8 hrly as required for fever
Refills: Nil

XY Jain
Stamp

Sample 2

Dr XY Jain
MBBS, MD (General Medicine)
Registration no. MPMC 223344
25, Park Street, Gwalior MP
Tel. no. 111222 Email: -------@-----.com

Date: 01.01.2021

Patient's name: Mr B
Age & Sex: Male
Address: 24, Modern Colony, Gwalior

Diagnosis: Acute Pharyngitis

R_x

Cap Amoxycillin/Clavulanic Acid (500/125 mg) orally 8 hrly for 5 days
Hot water gargles three times in a day

XY Jain
Stamp

Sample 3

Dr XY Jain
MBBS, MD (General Medicine)
Registration no. MPMC 223344
25, Park Street, Gwalior MP
Tel. no. 111222 Email: -------@-----.com

Date: 06.01.2021

Patient's name: Mr X
Age & Sex: 30 years, Male
Weight: 55 kg
Address: 24, Modern Colony, Gwalior

Diagnosis: Swine Flu

Tab Oseltamivir 75 mg orally 12 hrly for 5 days
Tab Paracetamol 500 mg 6–8 hrly as required for fever
Refills: None

XY Jain
Stamp

Sample 4

Dr XY Jain
MBBS, MD (General Medicine)
Registration no. MPMC 223344
25, Park Street, Gwalior MP
Tel. no. 111222 Email: -------@-----.com

Date: 07.01.2021

Patient's name: Mr B
Age & Sex: 50 years, Male
Weight: 55 kg
Address: 24, Modern Colony, Gwalior

Diagnosis: Intestinal Amoebiasis

R_X
Tab. Metronidazole 400 mg orally 8 hrly with meals
Refills: None

XY Jain
Stamp

Sample 5

Dr XY Jain
MBBS, MD (General Medicine)
Registration no. MPMC 223344
25, Park Street, Gwalior MP
Tel. no. 111222 Email: -------@-----.com

Date: 08.01.2021

Patient's name: Mr V
Age & Sex: 50 years, Male
Weight: 55 kg
Address: 24, Modern Colony, Gwalior

Diagnosis: Pseudomembranous Colitis

R_X
Flagyl 500 mg for 7 days
Refills: None

XY Jain
Stamp

Sample 6

Dr XY Jain
MBBS, MD (General Medicine)
Registration no. MPMC 223344
25, Park Street, Gwalior MP
Tel. no. 111222 Email: -------@-----.com

Date: 05.01.2021

Patient's name: Mr Y
Age & Sex: 50 years, Male
Weight: 55 kg
Address: 24, Modern Colony, Gwalior

Diagnosis: Pediculosis

R_X
Permethrin 1% lotion apply on dry hair
Allow to remain for 10 min then wash with water
Repeat after 7 days if lies detected

Sample 7

Dr XY Jain
MBBS, MD (General Medicine)
Registration no. MPMC 223344
25, Park Street, Gwalior MP
Tel. no. 111222 Email: -------@-----.com

Date: 08.01.2021

Patient's name: Mr B
Age & Sex: 50 years, Male
Weight: 55 kg
Address: 24, Modern Colony, Gwalior

Diagnosis: Iron Deficiency Anemia

R_X
Tab Ferrous Sulphate once a day

XY Jain
Stamp

Sample 8

Dr XY Jain
MBBS, MD (General Medicine)
Registration no. MPMC 223344
25, Park Street, Gwalior MP
Tel. no. 111222 Email: -------@-----.com

Date: 10.02.2021

Patient's name: Mr X
Age & Sex: 50 years, Male
Weight: 55 kg
Address: 24, Modern Colony, Gwalior

Diagnosis: *Pneumocystis jiroveci* Pneumonia

R_X
Tab Trimethoprim/Sulfamethoxazole (320/1600 mg) orally 8 hourly for 21 days
Tab Prednisolone 40 mg orally for 21 days
Refills: None

XY Jain
Stamp

Sample 9

Dr XY Jain
MBBS, MD (General Medicine)
Registration no. MPMC 223344
25, Park Street, Gwalior MP
Tel. no. 111222 Email: -------@-----.com

Date: 09.01.2021

Patient's name: Mr A
Age & Sex: 50 years, Male
Weight: 55 kg
Address: 24, Modern Colony, Gwalior

Diagnosis: Acne Vulgaris

R_X

Tab Tetracycline 250 mg 6 hrly orally with milk for 10 days

XY Jain
Stamp

Sample 10

Dr XY Jain
MBBS, MD (General Medicine)
Registration no. MPMC 223344
25, Park Street, Gwalior MP
Tel. no. 111222 Email: -------@-----.com

Date: 10.01.2021

Patient's name: Mr B
Age & Sex: 50 years, Male
Weight: 55 kg
Address: 24, Modern Colony, Gwalior

Diagnosis: Acute Bronchitis

R_X

Cap Amoxycillin 250 mg 8 hrly for 10 days
Tab Azithromycin 500 mg once daily for 3 days
Tab Paracetamol 500 mg 8 hrly for 10 days
Tab Cetirizine 10 mg once daily for 10 days
Tab Dexamethasone 0.5 mg once daily for 10 days
Tab B Complex once daily for 10 days
Cap Omeprazole 40 mg once daily for 10 days

XY Jain
Stamp

Sample 11

Dr XY Jain

MBBS, MD (General Medicine)

Registration no. MPMC 223344

25, Park Street, Gwalior MP

Tel. no. 111222 Email: -------@-----.com

Date: 02.02.2021

Patient's name: Mr X

Age & Sex: 50 years, Male

Weight: 55 kg

Address: 24, Modern Colony, Gwalior

Diagnosis: Toxoplasmosis

R_X

Tab Pyrimethamine 200 mg orally as first dose then 75 mg once daily for 6 weeks

Tab Sulfadiazine 1500 mg 6 hourly for 6 weeks

Tab folinic acid 10 mg orally once daily for 6 weeks

Tab Paracetamol 500 mg 8 hrly as required for fever

XY Jain

Stamp

Sample 12

Dr XY Jain

MBBS, MD (General Medicine)

Registration no. MPMC 223344

25, Park Street, Gwalior MP

Tel. no. 111222 Email: -------@-----.com

Date: 05.01.2021

Patient's name: Mr X

Age & Sex: 50 years, Male

Weight: 55 kg

Address: 24, Modern Colony, Gwalior

Diagnosis: Typhoid Fever

R_X

Tab Ciprofloxacin 750 mg BD for 14 days

Tab Paracetamol 500 mg SOS as required for fever

Tab Metoclopramide 10 mg TDS as required for vomiting

XY Jain

Stamp

Sample 13

Dr XY Jain
MBBS, MD (General Medicine)
Registration no. MPMC 223344
25, Park Street, Gwalior MP
Tel. no. 111222 Email: -------@-----.com

Date: 07.01.2021

Patient's name:
Age & Sex: 53 years, Male
Weight: 56 kg
Address: 24, Modern Colony, Gwalior

Diagnosis: Gonorrhoea

R_X

Inj Ceftriaxone 250 mg IM single dose
Tab Azithromycin 1 g single dose
Tab Paracetamol 500 mg 6–8 hrly as required for fever

XY Jain
Stamp

Sample 14

Dr XY Jain
MBBS, MD (General Medicine)
Registration no. MPMC 223344
25, Park Street, Gwalior MP
Tel. no. 111222 Email: -------@-----.com

Date: 02.01.2021

Patient's name: Mr A
Age & Sex: 30 years, Male
Weight: 59 kg
Address: 24, Modern Colony, Gwalior

Diagnosis: Roundworm Infestation

R_X

Tab Albendamol 400 mg single dose
Refills: None

XY Jain
Stamp

Sample 15

Dr XY Jain
MBBS, MD (General Medicine)
Registration no. MPMC 223344
25, Park Street, Gwalior MP
Tel. no. 111222 Email: -------@-----.com

Date: 06.01.2021

Patient's name: Ms V
Age & Sex: 28 years, Female
Weight: 58 kg
Address: 24, Modern Colony, Gwalior

Diagnosis: Acute Bronchitis in Pregnancy

R_X
Cap Doxycycline 100 mg 12 hrly orally on day 1 followed by 100 mg orally once daily for next 6 days

XY Jain
Stamp

Sample 16

Dr XY Jain
MBBS, MD (General Medicine)
Registration no. MPMC 223344
25, Park Street, Gwalior MP
Tel. no. 111222 Email: -------@-----.com

Date:

Patient's name: Mr A
Age & Sex: 28 years, Male
Address: 24, Modern Colony, Gwalior

Diagnosis: Upper Respiratory Tract Infection with Cough

R_X
Tab Erythromycin 500 mg orally 8 hrly for 5 days
Syrup Codeine Phosphate 5 mL orally 8 hrly for 5 days
Hot water gargles at 8 a.m., 2 p.m. and at 10 p.m. in a day for 5 days

XY Jain
Stamp

Errors Report and Correction Tips

Sample 1

Error report: Doctor's particulars like Doctor's name, professional degrees, and registration number, address and telephone number are missing. A doctor without a registration number is not authorized to write a prescription. This is a legal document. Without doctors details pharmacy personnel are in a dilemma whether the prescription is written by a registered practitioner or not. A pharmacist is not authorized to dispense drugs in such prescriptions and if he does so, he may be penalized. The patient cannot communicate with the doctor in case of any emergency.

Correction tips: Write doctor's particulars like doctor's name, professional degrees, address, telephone number and email address at the top of the prescription.

Sample 2

Error report: Patient's particulars like age and weight are missing. The age and weight of the patient are required to confirm appropriate doses of the drugs in the prescription. Patient's weight on the prescription can be useful in avoiding dosing errors, particularly when drugs are administered to paediatric patients. This also helps the pharmacy personnel to assess the prescription and be confident of dispensing the right drug and dosage form like syrup and not tablets for infants.

Correction tips: Write the patient's age and weight after the doctor's particulars.

Sample 3

Error report: Superscription symbol "R_X" is missing. This is a sign written in the name of God, which is universally accepted. It represents the specific Latin verb "recipe" which means "take thou". This symbol separates the superscription from inscription.

Correction tips: Write superscription symbol R_X just before inscription, on the left side.

Sample 4

Error report: Duration of treatment is missing. The patient is not advised for how long he needs to take the drugs for the cure of amoebiasis. If the patient leaves the treatment in between chances of recurrence will be there or the patient may take the drugs for longer than the required duration, result in ADR or increased cost to the patient.

Correction tips: In amoebiasis Tab Metronidazole is given in a dose of 400 mg orally 8 hrly for 10 days.

Sample 5

Error report: The dosage form of medicine is missing and the generic name of the drug is not used. What should be the route of administration is also not mentioned. The pharmacist may find it difficult to dispense the correct drug.

Correction tips: Right inscription for this patient of pseudomembranous colitis is: Tab Metronidazole 500 mg orally 8 hrly for 10 days.

Sample 6

Error report: The doctor's signature is missing. Without the signature of the prescribing physician, the prescription is not legal. The pharmacist cannot dispense drugs. Even if it is a computer typed prescription, it is considered illegal without the signature of prescribing doctor and drug addicts can misuse it. A prescription with a signature also rules out the possibility of photocopied or invalid prescription.

Correction tips: Add signature of the doctor below the inscription.

Sample 7

Error report: Instructions to the patient as to when to take the drug is missing. The patient should be instructed to take the drug after meals and not to worry if the colour of the stool is black. The strength of the drug is also not mentioned.

Correction tips: Write instructions and directions at the end of the prescription like take the drug after meals and colour of the stools may turn black because of iron. Also mention the dose of the drug—Tab Ferrous Sulfate 325 mg orally once daily after meals for one month.

Sample 8

Error report: How to taper steroids is not mentioned. Steroids should be tapered gradually and then stopped. If not withdrawn gradually it can result in exacerbation of the disease or acute adrenal insufficiency.

Correction tips: Correct way to prescribe steroid is:

Tab Prednisolone	40 mg 12 hourly for 5 days
	40 mg once daily for 5 days
	20 mg once daily for 11 days

Sample 9

Error report: Preferred dosage form is a capsule, not tablet because tetracycline has irritant property can cause epigastric pain, nausea and diarrhoea. Tetracycline is not to be given with milk because of its chelating property. It forms an insoluble and unabsorbable complex with calcium. If given with milk may lead to treatment failure on account of lesser drug absorption from the gut.

Correction tips: Ideally the tetracycline capsule should be taken two hours before or two hours after food. It should not be given with milk and dairy products.

Add supplemental instructions: When prescribing tetracycline, the patient should be warned to avoid sun exposure to prevent photoallergy.

Sample 10

Error report: The inscription part is not as per guidelines. Polypharmacy is there. Polypharmacy is defined as the use of five or more medications daily by an individual.

Correction tips: Only cap Amoxycillin 500 mg orally 8 hrly and tab Paracetamol 500 mg as required for fever are sufficient.

Sample 11

Error report: Prescription is not legible as it is written in bad handwriting. It may create confusion and increase the chances of errors. There are chances of wrong drugs being dispensed as the pharmacist may use guesswork.

Correction tips: The inscription part of this prescription should be written in clear handwriting or it should be typed.

Tab Pyrimethamine 200 mg orally as the first dose then 75 mg once daily for 6 weeks
Tab Sulfadiazine 1500 mg 6 hourly for 6 weeks
Tab Folinic Acid 10 mg orally once daily for 6 weeks
Tab Paracetamol 500 mg 8 hrly as required for fever

Sample 12

Error report: One very common cause of prescription errors is the use of abbreviations for the frequency of administration as OD, BD, TDS or SOS. These abbreviations can be misinterpreted by the patients not knowing Latin. It is recommended that abbreviations are not to be used at all when writing medication orders.

Correction tips: Frequency of administration is to be written as:

Tab Ciprofloxacin 750 mg 12 hourly for 7 days
Tab Paracetamol 500 mg orally 6 hrly as required for fever
Tab Metoclopramide 10 mg 8 hrly before meals as required for vomiting

Sample 13

Error report: Name of the patient is missing. If the name of the patient is not mentioned, the prescription cannot be linked to a particular patient with certainty. Complete name of the patient must be written. A prescription is meant for an individual and if the half name is written there may be two clients at the pharmacy with the same first/last names whose prescriptions may get interchanged therefore along with the complete name, patient's age and address are important for proper identification of a patient.

Correction tips: Write the complete name of the patient.

Sample 14

Error report: The spelling of the drug's name is wrong. There is a chance for error by pharmacist and wrong drug may be dispensed or pharmacist may refuse to dispense the drug.

Correction tips: The spelling of the drug name should be correct.

Tab Albendazole 400 mg orally single dose.

Sample 15

Error report: Tetracyclines are contraindicated in pregnancy as they have an affinity with calcium. They are taken up by the growing teeth and bone of the fetus. They should not be prescribed for pregnant patients because of their potential for permanent discoloration of teeth in the fetus (yellow or brown in appearance), as well as impairment of fetal long bone growth.

Correction tips: A drug that is safe in pregnancy is to be prescribed.
Cap Amoxycillin 500 mg 8 hourly for 5 days.

Sample 16

Error report: Date of prescription is missing. In this prescription Codeine syrup is advised for cough which is a drug of dependence. The patient may misuse this prescription to purchase Codeine syrup several times in absence of mention of date on the prescription. The prescriber has also not given required important directions to the dispenser about refills. Writing of date is very important for medicolegal cases.

Correction tips: To write the date of prescription and direction to the dispenser.
"Not to refill until instructed".

Chapter 5

Prescribing for Special Groups

Dose adjustments are required when there is a change in physiology and/or associated pathology in an individual on the account of changes in pharmacokinetics and pharmacodynamics of drugs.

Prescription writing must be appropriate and meticulous as per individual. To write correct doses in these different conditions are an important part of prescribing skill.

PRESCRIBING IN PAEDIATRICS

Infants and children are not small adults. Just by a proportionate reduction in adult dose, the optimum paediatric dose cannot be obtained. Paediatric prescribing is much more complicated than adult prescribing for a number of reasons:

- Pharmacokinetics and pharmacodynamics are different in children and they also vary between different age groups.
- Clinical trials are rarely conducted in children; so many drugs are used off label.
- Special methods of drug administration are required for infants and young children, e.g. solid dosage forms like tablets, capsules or metered dose inhalers are difficult to administer in infants.
- Dose calculations are required and any error in calculation can be more serious than in adults.

Classification of Pediatric Patients

- *Neonate:* Birth to 28 days
- *Infant:* 29 days to one year
- *Toddler:* 1 to 3 years
- *Young child:* 3 to 5 years
- *Older child:* 6 to 12 years
- *Adolescent:* 13 to 18 years

What is different in paediatric pharmacokinetics?

With the developmental changes from neonate to adolescence, there are changes in the absorption, distribution, metabolism and excretion of medications in children.

Drug Absorption

Gut transit time is slow and gastric acid level is low in children as compared to adults. The absorption of ampicillin is more efficient in neonates than in adults because of the higher gastric pH.

Systemic absorption across the skin surface is prompt because the skin is thin and permeable to drugs.

Milk in the stomach can influence the oral absorption of drugs in neonates and infants.

Rectal absorption is very efficient in neonates, e.g. diazepam solution is given per rectally to control febrile seizures in children less than 5 years of age.

IM route should be avoided because of less muscle mass, less blood supply and more pain.

Drug Distribution

Body composition of water and fat content is different in neonates. A neonate has more total body water than fat that decreases with age. The volume of distribution is therefore increased for water-soluble drugs so higher doses of water-soluble drugs are required than adults.

Blood–brain barrier is more permeable to drugs allowing higher concentration in CNS.

Plasma protein concentrations are lower in neonates so plasma protein binding of drugs is low, this results in a higher unbound fraction of the drug and increased chances of adverse effects, e.g. warfarin.

Drug Biotransformation

Different enzyme systems in the liver mature at different rates, overall metabolism is lower in neonates. Gray baby syndrome with chloramphenicol is seen as the enzyme glucuronyl transferase for phase II reactions is not adequately formed. Drugs like diazepam, nalidixic acid, lignocaine and succinylcholine act longer because they are poorly metabolised. Enzymes maturation increases to adult levels in the first few months and then exceeds adult rates for the majority of childhood.

Drug Excretion

Kidney function matures by the age of 6–8 months. At birth, a newborn has 33% of the GFR and renal tubular excretion capacities of an adult so doses of drugs dependent on renal excretion such as aminoglycosides and penicillins must be adjusted in a neonate. Plasma half-lives of such drugs are increased by 3 to 5 times.

What is different in paediatric pharmacodynamics?

Because children do not have fully developed receptor and neurotransmitter systems hence the pharmacodynamic responses are not the same as in the adults. Some differences in drug actions also exist such as barbiturates which produce sedation in adults may produce excitation in children.

Selecting Doses of Medicine and Regimens in Children

Similar principles apply for selecting medicines for children as do for adults, but it is even more important to ensure that drug therapy is really needed that too in appropriate doses. Recommendations of dosage in the package insert by drug manufacturers are considered as reliable information. The prescriber can also refer national formulary for paediatric dosage. However, such information is not available for most of the drugs because children are not included in dose optimization studies. There are various formulas to calculate a child's dose from an adult's dose based on age, weight or body surface area. The most accurate method is the calculation of a child's dose using body surface area because the metabolic rate, redistribution of drugs, blood volume, extracellular fluid volume and renal blood flow all are closely related to it.

Age Based Calculation

Young's Formula; for Children 2 Years and Older

$$\text{Dose in child} = \frac{\text{Age in years}}{\text{Age} + 12} \times \text{Adult dose}$$

Fried's Formula; for Children up to 2 Years of Age

$$\text{Dose in child} = \frac{\text{Age in months}}{150} \times \text{Adult dose}$$

Dilling's Formula

$$\text{Dose in child} = \frac{\text{Age in years}}{20} \times \text{Adult dose}$$

Weight Based Calculation

Clark's Formula

$$\text{Dose in child} = \frac{\text{Body wt in kg}}{70} \times \text{Adult dose}$$

Body Surface Area Based Calculation

$$\text{Dose in child} = \frac{\text{BSA }(\text{m}^2)}{1.73\ (\text{m}^2)} \times \text{Adult dose}$$

Table 5.1: Body surface area (BSA) of children

Age	*Ideal body weight in kg*	*BSA (m^2)*	*% of adult dose*
Newborn	3.2	0.23	12.5
1 month	4	0.26	15
3 months	5.5	0.32	18
6 months	7.5	0.4	22
1 year	10	0.47	25
3 years	14	0.62	33
5 years	18	0.73	40
7 years	23	0.88	50
12 years	37	1.25	75

Table 5.2: Drugs not safe in children

Name of drug	*Adverse effects*
Tetracyclines	Growth retardation, teeth discoloration
Corticosteroids	Growth retardation
Androgens	Stunting of stature
Aspirin	Rey's syndrome
Chloramphenicol	Gray baby syndrome
Sulphonamides	Jaundice
Fluoroquinolones	Arthropathy
Phenothiazines	Dystonia
Metoclopramide	Acute dystonia

Body surface area can be calculated by Dubois formula

BSA (m^2) = BW (kg)$^{0.425}$ × Height (cm)$^{0.725}$ × 0.007184

PRESCRIBING IN ELDERLY

The elderly means persons more than 65 years of age. Currently, they represent about 10% of the Indian population. Prescribing in the elderly is challenging because

- The elderly persons experience a greater incidence of diseases and physical impairments than younger adults, e.g. impaired memory, impaired eyesight, immobility, lethargy and tremors in hand.
- The elderly suffers more from adverse drug effects and drug-drug interactions than younger adults because of impairment of homeostatic mechanisms and the effects of coexisting diseases.
- Compliance is poor in the elderly may be due to impaired hearing, several drugs, complex drug regimen, etc.
- Polypharmacy is a common problem amongst elderly people and the degree of polypharmacy increases with the advancing age.
- Vitamins, minerals and nutrients deficiencies are more common in elderly.
- Coexisting diseases like hypertension and diabetes mellitus lead to renal compromise.

What is different in geriatric pharmacokinetics?

Physiological changes caused by ageing vary among patients and should be considered before prescribing.

Drug Absorption

The absorption rate of drugs is reduced in the elderly due to reduced gut motility and blood flow to the intestine, with a longer time needed to reach peak concentrations.

First Pass Metabolism

Normally drugs are first absorbed from the gut and then metabolised in the liver before reaching the systemic circulation. In elderly people first pass metabolism may be reduced because of decreased liver mass and blood flow. This means that drugs that would normally undergo significant initial metabolism will have higher bioavailability, e.g. propranolol, labetalol, verapamil, metoclopramide, opioids and diazepam.

Prodrugs which require metabolism to change from an inactive to active form will have lower bioavailability.

Drug Distribution

Drug distribution can be affected by the changes in body composition, i.e. proportionally less muscle mass and total body water and more body fat in the elderly. This can affect the volume of distribution, which may result in either increased plasma concentrations or half-life of some drugs causing toxicity, e.g. digoxin and lithium. Protein binding may also change causing an increase in the free fraction of highly bound acidic drugs and a possible decrease in the free fraction of basic drugs, e.g. Plasma protein binding of warfarin may decrease.

Drug Excretion

As the age advances there is a reduction in GFR by 6–10% every 10 years after the age of 40 years. At least a 50% reduction in GFR is seen by the age of 70 years. Creatinine clearance is markedly reduced in the elderly, so drugs doses have to be reduced, e.g. Streptomycin 0.75 g after 50 years of age and 0.5 g after 70 years of age is prescribed as compared to young adults requiring 1 g. Renal plasma flow and active secretion of drugs may decrease so excretion of renally cleared drugs may decrease, e.g. digoxin, lithium, penicillin, vancomycin.

What is different in Geriatric Pharmacodynamics?

- The number of receptors and binding to receptors decrease in the elderly, e.g. beta receptors sensitivity to both agonist and antagonist is reduced.
- Receptor response to CNS depressant drugs is increased, e.g. morphine, diazepam.
- Reduction in baroreceptor reflex sensitivity is seen so chances of postural hypotension are increased with agents that lower blood pressure.
- Augmented effects like hypovolemia and electrolyte disturbances are seen with diuretics and hypoglycemia with antidiabetics.

Tips for Safe Prescribing in the Elderly

When prescribing in the elderly, consider the following:

- Make sure whether drug therapy is a suitable therapeutic option or a non-pharmacological approach might be better. If drug therapy is necessary the dosage should be titrated to a clearly defined goal starting from a low initial dose.
- When initiating a new medication in elderly patients choose agents with known pharmacokinetic properties.
- In order to enhance patient compliance prescribe the drugs with less frequent dosing especially at the time of discharge from hospital.
- In the case of comorbidities when more than two or three drugs are to be given try to avoid drugs that are inhibitors or inducers of cytochrome P450 hepatic metabolism enzymes or are highly plasma protein bound, e.g. valproic acid, phenytoin ceftriaxone, diazepam and warfarin.
- When the maintenance dose of a medication is not established, increase the dose gradually to achieve a desired clinical effect.

- Maintenance doses of renally excreted drugs, e.g. digoxin should be lower than usual.
- Whenever an elderly patient develops a new or unexplained medical problem after drug intake, consider adverse drug reaction as a cause, e.g. delirium, hypotension, arrhythmias, renal failure, electrolyte disorders and constipation.
- Be clear about the diagnosis. Take care not to prescribe a drug to manage an adverse effect from another drug unless this is unavoidable.
- Think about whether the drug you are considering causes a particular problem in the elderly patients or has a narrow safety margin, e.g. warfarin. Can it be safely used in this patient?
- While treating elderly patients it is always needed to check that the drugs prescribed are appropriate to achieve the aim and if not, stop them. Properly communicate with the patient and family after reviewing the medications and provide written directions.
- Considering old age problems like forgetfulness and difficulty in opening the packaging, keep the drug regimens as simple as possible.

One should not deny prescribing beneficial medicines to elderly patients just because they are old. Since clinical trials are not performed in elderly patients so there is a chance that the use of drugs may not provide the same benefit to the old age group as in the younger population.

Precaution While Using Certain Medicines in Elderly Patients

Some drugs are more challenging to use in elderly patients and some are best avoided altogether.

Hypnotics

Benzodiazepines should not be routinely prescribed for insomnia. Increased sensitivity to benzodiazepines is well recognized with increasing age and also there is a possible increase in half-life, both of which contribute to 'hangover' effects seen the next day. Elderly patients are at increased risk of falls and cognitive impairment. If a benzodiazepine must be used, choose one with a short half-life such as lorazepam and use it for the shortest possible time.

Neuroleptic Drugs

Neuroleptic drugs, often prescribed for agitation in the elderly, can cause delirium, extrapyramidal symptoms and postural hypotension in the short-term and possibly stroke in the long-term. Avoid these drugs if possible and consider other non-pharmacological measures.

Analgesics

Opioid sensitivity is increased in the elderly as is a reduction in clearance. Initial doses of 25 to 50% of normal adult doses are recommended in the elderly. Tramadol works on serotonin and adrenergic receptors as well as opioid ones, giving it a different side-effect profile. This includes a reduced seizure threshold and delirium, which may make it less useful in the elderly. Pethidine should also be avoided.

Nonsteroidal anti-inflammatory drugs (NSAIDs) pose particular problems in the elderly. There is a greater risk of gastrointestinal, cardiovascular and renal adverse effects. These drugs should be avoided where possible, and, if used should be for the shortest possible time with the lowest possible dose and close monitoring.

Digoxin

Digoxin has a narrow therapeutic index and its pharmacokinetics are altered in the elderly (decreased volume of distribution, reduced clearance), making toxicity a potential problem. Both loading and maintenance doses should be reduced, with a maximum maintenance dose of 125 micrograms (half of the normal maximum dose).

Anticoagulants

Elderly patients are more sensitive to the effects of warfarin, and at greater risk of adverse effects. However, it is also often omitted unnecessarily in elderly patients with atrial fibrillation who may benefit from it. Particular risks may be: Possible interactions with antiplatelet drugs, gastrointestinal bleeding and tendency to fall of patients. If warfarin is used, lower loading and maintenance doses are recommended.

Antihypertensive Drugs

Elderly patients have a lower resting heart rate and decreased tachycardic response to postural changes. They are therefore more susceptible to the bradycardiac and hypotensive effects of many drugs. Angiotensin-converting enzyme inhibitors are less useful in the elderly and may cause increased renal impairment. Calcium channel blockers may contribute to constipation. Both verapamil and diltiazem have increased antihypertensive effects in the elderly.

Anticholinergic Drugs

Many drug classes have anticholinergic effects (e.g. antihistamines, antidepressants and neuroleptics) that can be more pronounced in the elderly. Urinary retention, constipation and postural hypotension can be more problematic in the elderly. Try to avoid multiple anticholinergics in combination.

Antibiotics

Antibiotic associated diarrhoea and *Clostridium difficile* infection are more common in the elderly. Some other adverse effects of antibiotics like delirium, seizures, haematological abnormalities and renal damage are also more common in the elderly than in younger patients.

PRESCRIBING IN PREGNANCY

To balance the risks and benefits of drug therapy during pregnancy is a challenge for every clinician because pharmacokinetic and pharmacodynamic processes are altered by pregnancy and any drug administered to a pregnant woman may harm the developing fetus or influence her pregnancy adversely.

However, pharmacological treatment is unavoidable in pregnancy with some medical conditions, e.g. asthma, epilepsy and hypertension to prevent complications in the mother.

Pharmacokinetic Changes during Pregnancy

Absorption: Gastric tone and motility are decreased, which result in a delay in the GI emptying time and absorption of drugs given orally.

Volume of distribution: Plasma volume increases approximately 50% of normal by 24 to 28 weeks gestation, increasing the volume of distribution so drugs may require dosage adjustments.

Protein binding: The blood volume increases in pregnancy due to the increase in free water. This in turn results in dilution of plasma proteins and increased free drug levels for a particular total serum level.

Hepatic clearance: In pregnancy quite often hepatic clearance of drugs increases.

Renal clearance: There is about a 50% increase in glomerular filtration rate in pregnancy from the normal range, so many drugs that are renally cleared require dosage alterations in pregnancy, for example, digoxin doses may need to be increased in the second trimester.

Pharmacodynamic Changes in Pregnancy

Changes do occur in receptor function and blood flow to tissues but clinical implications are not clear.

Placental Transfer of Drugs

The placenta is the functional unit formed by the chorionic villi of the embryo and the decidua basalis of the endometrium of the uterus of the mother.

Important functions of the placenta include respiration, nutrition, metabolism, excretion and endocrine activity to maintain fetal wellbeing. Drugs may cause pharmacological or teratogenic effects in the embryo or fetus, by crossing the maternal circulation to the fetal circulation or tissues via the placenta.

Factors Responsible for Placental Drug Transfer

Physicochemical properties of a drug affect placental transfer such as:
Molecular weight: Drugs with low molecular weight (less than 500 daltons) diffuse freely across the placenta than high molecular weight drugs (500–1000 daltons). Very large molecular weight drugs, e.g. heparins do not cross the placental membranes.

pH: Weakly acidic and weakly basic drugs diffuse across the placental membranes.

Lipid solubility: Lipid-soluble drugs easily diffuse across the placental membranes.

Plasma protein binding: Unbound free drug crosses the placenta.

Physical characteristics of the placenta: With the progress of pregnancy the placental membranes become progressively thinner, resulting in a decrease in diffusion distance.

In diseases of the mother like maternal hypertension or diabetes there may be reduced or enhanced placental drug transfer.

General Principles of Prescribing in Pregnancy

- Avoid medications in the first trimester as far as possible.
- Inform prospective parents fully and take their consent in the decision-making process.

- Consider the risk of relapse against potential adversity to fetus and mother.
- Use those drugs that are effective at minimal doses and avoid drugs which have demonstrated evidence of harm to the fetus during pregnancy, e.g. sodium valproate.
- Keep in mind the changes in pharmacokinetics with the progress of the pregnancy while prescribing drugs. Dosing intervals may need to be shortened in pregnancy. For example, once a day agent to control blood pressure may not be enough and dosing frequency may have to be increased for adequate control of blood pressure.
- Periodic monitoring of drug levels should be done before adjusting doses. Instead of total serum levels, free drug levels are better guides.

Effects of drugs on pregnancy: In general congenital anomalies occur in 2–4% of all live births.

Table 5.3: Gestational stages: Drug effects

Stage	*Duration*	*Effects*
Preimplantation stage	15 days from conception to implantation	Abortion/not affecting at all
Period of organogenesis	from 17th to 56th day	Abortion Congenital malformations
Second and third trimester	From 91 days onwards	Congenital malformations Retardation of growth behavioral Abnormality premature labor Neonatal toxicity Postnatal effects, e.g. tetracyclines
During labour	At term	Neonatal toxicity, e.g. opioids

Table 5.4: FDA pregnancy categories of drug use

The FDA has a categorization of drug risks to the fetus that runs from: "Category A" (safest) to "Category X" (known danger—do not use)

Category	*Risk*	*Drugs*
A	No fetal risk in controlled human studies	Folic acid Thyroxine
B	Animal studies show fetal risk but human studies do not show risk	Metronidazole Meclizine
C	Animal reproduction studies have shown an adverse effect on the fetus and there are no adequate and well-controlled studies in humans. Risk cannot be ruled out. Potential benefits may warrant the use of the drug in pregnant women despite potential risks	Corticosteroids Tramadol Gabapentin Amlodipine Trazodone
D	Positive fetal risk in human. Potential benefits may warrant use of the drug in pregnant women despite potential risks (e.g., if the drug is needed in a life-threatening situation or for a serious disease for which safer drugs cannot be used or are ineffective)	Antiepileptics Lisinopril Losartan Alprazolam Clonazepam Lorazepam
X	Studies in animals or humans have demonstrated fetal abnormalities. The risks involved in the use of the drug in pregnant women clearly outweigh potential benefits	Cytotoxic drugs

Out of all birth defects, only 3% are ascribed to drugs/environmental factors/radiation/maternal infection

The harmful effects on the fetus depend upon:

- Stage of gestation at which the drug is used
- Nature of drug
- Dose of drug
- Genetic constitution and susceptibility of the fetus
- Age and health of the mother

The greatest risk to the fetus is from the third to the eleventh week of pregnancy. During the second and third trimester drugs may affect the growth and functional development of the fetus.

Drugs given shortly before labor may have adverse effects on neonate after birth.

Table 5.5: Drugs in category X

Class of drugs	*Characteristic abnormalities*
Anticancer drugs	Abortion, various malformations, CNS and limb abnormalities
Retinoids (etretinate, isotretinoin)	Skeletal and cerebral abnormalities
Thalidomide	Phocomelia
Warfarin	Hydroencephaly, microcephaly, nasal hypoplasia and skeletal defects
Misoprostol	Möbius syndrome
Oestrogen	Feminization of male fetus, vaginal carcinoma of female offspring
Androgen	Masculinization of female fetus
Danazol	Masculinization of female fetus

Table 5.6: Drugs in category D

Class of drugs	*Characteristic abnòrmalities*
Tetracycline	Anomalies of teeth and bone
Streptomycin	Ototoxicity
Penicillamine	Cutis laxa and other malformations
Lisinopril, Losartan	Fetal hypotension, renal dysfunction
Alprazolam, Clonazepam	Cleft lip, cleft palate

Table 5.7: Effects of drugs during late trimester

Drugs	*Effects*
Sex hormones	Masculinization
Antithyroid drugs	Foetal goiter
Tetracyclines	Tooth and bone development
Corticosteroids	Growth retardation
NSAIDs, e.g. aspirin, indomethacin	Early closure of ductus arteriosus
	Onset of labor is delayed, impaired CNS development

Table 5.8: Drugs apparently safe in pregnancy

S.no.	*Ailment*	*Drugs*
1	Nausea and vomiting	Cyclizine, Meclizine, Diphenhydramine, Dimenhydrinate, Metoclapramide can be used in third trimester
2	Heartburn	Nonsystemic antacids
3	Peptic ulcer	Sucralfate, H2 receptor blockers, Bismuth Subsalicylate
4	Constipation	Milk of magnesia, Docusate sodium, Glycerin, Bisacodyl
5	Tuberculosis	Isoniazid, Ethambutol, Rifampicin
6	Amoebiasis	Metronidazole, Diodoquin, Diloxanide
7	Worm infestation	Piperazine citrate, Pyrantel pamoate, Niclosamide, Bephenium hydroxynaphthoate, Praziquantel
8	Malaria	Chloroquine, Quinine, Proguanil, Pyrimethamine are safe, whereas Mefloquine, Artemether and Lumefantrine (safe in 2nd and 3rd trimester)
9	Hypertension	Methyl-Dopa, Labetalol
10	Heart disease	Treated as in nonpregnant women (Digoxin, Quinidine, β-blocker)
11	Thromboembolism	Heparin (unfractionated)
12	Allergic rhinitis	*Local* (Glucocorticoids and Decongestants) Systemic: Antihistaminics-diphenhydramine, Dimenhydrinate
13	Dry cough	Diphenhydramine, Codeine, Dextromethorphan
14	Pruritus	*Local* (Calamine lotion, Zinc oxide cream or ointment, Glucocorticoid) *Systemic* (Hydroxizine, Diphenhydramine, Glucocorticoids)
15	Headache	Paracetamol, Aspirin and NSAIDs (only in 1st 2nd trimester)
16	Migraine	Analgesics, Propranolol, Dimenhydrinate, Amitriptyline
17	Bronchial asthma	Inhaled Adrenergic agonists, inhaled Glucocorticoids, Aminophylline
18	Diabetes mellitus	Insulin
19	Thyrotoxicosis	Thioamides (Propylthiouracil preferred to Carbimazole/ Methimazole)
20	Hypothyroidism	Thyroxine
21	Epilepsy	Phenobarbitone, Carbamazepine; folic acid and vitamin K1
22	Depression/ psychosis/anxiety	Phenothiazines, TCAs, SSRI (except Paroxetine), Diazepam
23	General anaesthesia	Thiopentone sodium, Nitrous oxide
24	Infections	Penicillins, Cephalosporins, Erythromycin base, Nitrofurantoin, Methanamine mandelate, Metronidazole (anaerobic infections), Aminoglycosides (only Gentamicin or Tobramycin preferred if serious systemic infection to be treated)
25	Fungal infection	Miconazole, Clotrimazole, Nystatin, Tolnaftate
26	Viral infection	Acyclovir (used only if potential benefit outweighs the risk)
27	HIV infection	Zidovudine, Lamivudine, Stavudine, Nevirapine, Nelfinavir, Saquinavir. Zidovudine + lamivudine + Nevirapine (to prevent perinatal transmission)

PRESCRIBING IN LACTATION

In mothers who are breastfeeding, consideration of whether the child will be exposed to the drug, and what consequences this may have, is important. Unfortunately, data on these aspects may not be available because of the lack of clinical trial in breastfeeding patients. Most data comes from observational studies, and so there may be more information about older drugs.

Many substances ingested by lactating women are present in breast milk, although the levels tend to be less than *in utero*. It is important to know both the likely concentration and the potential effects in order to estimate risk. Toxicity to infant can occur if the drug enters the milk in significant quantities. The concentration of some drugs in milk may exceed that in the maternal plasma, e.g. iodides so that the therapeutic dose in the mother can cause toxicity to the infant.

Some drugs may inhibit the suckling reflex in infants, e.g. phenobarbitone.

Selecting Medicines and Regimes in Breastfeeding

In general, drugs that are safe in children under two years of age are safe in breast feeding, but if possible choose drugs that are present in breast milk at lower concentrations.

Drugs that decrease serum prolactin levels
- Ergot alkaloids
- L-dopa
- Bromocriptine

Drugs that increase serum prolactin levels
- Metoclopramide
- Methyldopa
- Amphetamines
- Haloperidol
- Phenothiazine
- Theophylline

Table 5.9: Drugs contraindicated during lactation

Examples	*Adverse effects on breastfed babies*
Anticancer drugs	Impaired growth, carcinogenesis and immunosuppression
Radioactive drugs	Carcinogenesis
Chloramphenicol	Bone marrow suppression
Etretinate	Hepatotoxicity
Mesoprostol	Diarrhoea
Carbimazole and methimazole	Hypothyroidism
Lovastatin	Hepatotoxicity
Lithium	Hypotonia, bradycardia and thyroid dysfunction
Amiodarone	Thyroid dysfunction
Warfarin	Bleeding
ACE inhibitors	Hypotension
Amphetamine and methamphetamine	Insomnia, CNS stimulant effect

Drugs that readily enter breast milk
- Narcotics
- Barbiturates
- Benzodiazepine
- Antidepressants
- Antipsychotics
- Metoclopramide
- Anticholinergic

PRESCRIBING IN HEPATIC DISEASE

The liver plays an important role in the interactions between drugs and the body. That is why knowledge of the hepatic function of a patient is required for safe prescribing.

What is different about patients with liver disease?

The liver is the major organ involved in the metabolism of drugs. In addition, pharmacokinetic and pharmacodynamic processes are also altered in liver disease. The main changes in pharmacokinetics and pharmacodynamics in liver disease are as follows.

Impaired Absorption

Bioavailability of lipid soluble drugs may be reduced in cholestasis.

Impaired Drug Distribution

Hypoalbuminaemia is a feature of severe liver disease, where the amount of albumin available for drug binding is less. This in turn affects plasma protein binding of drugs so the unbound drug concentration increases, e.g. warfarin. Toxicity may occur with highly protein bound drugs having a narrow therapeutic index (e.g. phenytoin).

Impaired Metabolism

Liver disease may reduce the capacity to metabolise certain drugs leading to toxicity. This is caused by both the reduction in the metabolic capacity of the liver and the changes in liver blood flow. The dose of drugs that have a high hepatic extraction ratio (high first pass metabolism) needs to be reduced. On the other hand, prodrugs, e.g. captopril might become ineffective.

Impaired Excretion

In hepatobiliary disease, the biliary system is obstructed affecting excretion of some medicines and may lead to accumulation of drugs and toxicity. Renal impairment can also occur as a consequence of liver disease, e.g. in cirrhosis there is a reduction in glomerular filtration rate so dose adjustment is important for renally cleared drugs.

Altered Pharmacodynamics

Complications of liver disease such as hepatic encephalopathy, ascites and deficiencies in clotting factors can increase sensitivity to particular drug effects. Drugs that cause sedation, constipation or hypokalaemia, if given in severe liver disease can cause encephalopathy. Drugs that cause fluid retention, e.g. nonsteroidal anti-inflammatory drugs and prednisolone if given in ascitic patients may worsen it. Anticoagulants will require careful monitoring and adjustment in severe liver disease as clotting factors are usually depleted.

Hepatotoxicity Caused by Drugs

Many medicines can cause liver damage, through a wide range of mechanisms including hepatitis, cholestasis, nonalcoholic steatohepatitis and cirrhosis. Theoretically, such drugs should be avoided wherever possible in patients with liver disease to prevent further hepatic impairment; however, it has been argued that in practice most medications can be used safely in patients with chronic hepatic impairment because the liver has a large reserve capacity. Important exceptions include methotrexate in patients with alcoholic liver disease, and antitubercular drugs and antihuman immunodeficiency virus drugs in patients with hepatitis B or C.

Points to be considered while Selecting Medicines and Regimens in Liver Disease

As with all medicines, it is important to consider the risks and benefits of treatment in each patient. There is no well-accepted method of judging the degree of liver impairment, unlike in renal impairment, when making prescribing decisions. Raised liver enzymes indicate hepatic impairment but do not help to know about exact pathology. If possible, hepatotoxic drugs and drugs that may worsen the patient's clinical condition should be avoided.

- For drugs that are extensively hepatically metabolised, it may be considered in terms of whether it has a narrow or wide therapeutic index (i.e. the difference between the effective and toxic doses). Drugs with a narrow therapeutic index should be avoided and if at all to be used it should be used with extreme caution, e.g. theophylline should be given in less than 50% of the normal loading and maintenance dose.

  Drugs with a wide therapeutic index may be used with a reduced dose or frequency of administration. It is also to be kept in mind that even medicines that are only partially metabolised in the liver may become toxic at normal doses in severe liver disease.
- It is also important to consider what type of liver disease the patient has. Absorption of drugs is decreased in cholestatic disease, whereas biliary excretion of drugs is decreased in hepatocellular disease.
- Drugs that can cause renal impairment should also be used with care in liver disease because of the danger of hepatorenal syndrome. As the liver has considerable reserve so problems with drug use are visible only in severe disease. Estimation of liver impairment is also challenging because the liver has large reserve capacity and it is difficult to predict what will happen in a particular individual. For dose adjustment in liver disease, there is no endogenous marker.
- Drugs with narrow therapeutic index and low hepatic extraction or high bioavailability.

Common Drugs to be used with Caution in Hepaic Diseases

- *Paracetamol:* Can be given but lower doses are recommended, including for patients with excess alcohol intake who do not have proven alcoholic liver disease.

- *Aspirin and NSAIDs:* Because synthesis of clotting factors from liver is decreased, there is increased risk of bleeding with aspirin, whereas fluid and water retention with NSAIDs can increase ascites.
- *Anticoagulants:* Synthesis of clotting factors is reduced so the effect of warfarin may increase. Thrombin inhibitors may increase bleeding risk in liver disease for similar reasons.
- *Antidiabetic drugs:* There is an increased risk of lactic acidosis with metformin therapy. An increased risk of hypoglycemia is seen with sulphonylureas. Glitazones should be avoided because of the potential for hepatotoxicity.
- *Opiates and benzodiazepines:* May precipitate encephalopathy.

Drugs to be used with Reduced Dosage in Hepatic Impairment

Erythromycin, propranolol, rifampicin, cefoperazone, theophylline, colchicine, doxycycline, ethionamide, clonazepam, clindamycin, griseofulvin, metoprolol acebutolol INH, mercaptopurine, heparin and warfarin.

PRESCRIBING IN RENAL DISEASE

The kidney is the main organ for the elimination of drugs from the body. The number of patients with chronic kidney disease and reduced renal functions is increasing so it is important to learn dose adjustment for safe prescribing in patients with renal disease.

What is different about patients with renal disease?

The most important organ involved in the excretion of drugs is the kidney. If there is a decrease in glomerular filtration rate (GFR) there is a decrease in effective drug clearance. Pharmacokinetic and pharmacodynamic changes are also seen in renal diseases that require alteration in dosing.

Impaired Distribution

Protein binding of drugs may be altered because of hypoalbuminaemia (caused by proteinuria) or uraemia. Highly protein bound drugs with narrow therapeutic index are likely to cause toxicity due to reductions in protein binding.

Impaired Metabolism

Certain drugs are metabolized in the kidney and may be affected by various types of renal diseases. Drug metabolism in the liver tends to be slower in chronic renal disease. Many active metabolites of drugs depend on the kidney for their removal. They increase in renal impairment thereby increasing the incidence of ADR.

Impaired Excretion

The kidney excretes drugs through the processes of glomerular filtration, active tubular secretion and passive tubular reabsorption. All these functions are reduced in renal disease. Drugs that are renally cleared may require dose adjustment or avoidance.

Pharmacodynamic Changes

Sensitivity to certain drugs is altered in renal diseases leading to various adverse drug effects.

Nephrotoxicity by Drugs

Many commonly used drugs are nephrotoxic at intrinsic or post-renal levels. Many drugs cause intrinsic renal damage by acute tubular necrosis or acute interstitial nephritis. Post-renal obstruction can be occasionally drug induced. Nephrotoxic drugs should be avoided if possible in patients with renal disease as they may cause a further reduction in renal function. Examples of nephrotoxic drugs include: Aminoglycosides, amphotericin B, NSAIDs, sulphonamides and cyclosporine.

Selecting Doses of Medicines and Regimens in Renal Disease

The decline in functions of the kidney in a disease requires dose adjustment which can be calculated by:

$$\text{Dose in renal disease} = \frac{\text{Patient's creatinine clearance} \times \text{Normal dose}}{\text{Normal creatinine clearance}}$$

Creatinine clearance (mL/min) is the quantitative indicator of renal function which is calculated by Cockroft Gault's formula: Applicable to patients between the age of 40–80.

Creatinine (Cr) clearance (mL/min) for male

$$\frac{140 - \text{Age (years)} \times \text{Weight (kg)}}{72 \times \text{Serum Cr (mg/dL)}}$$

Creatinine (Cr) clearance (mL/min) for female

$$\frac{140\text{–Age (years)} \times \text{Weight (kg)}}{72 \times \text{Serum Cr (mg/dL)}} \times 0.85$$

Stages of Renal Impairment

Classification of renal function is important for prescribing guidance and is normally approximated by the GFR as defined by creatinine clearance.

Prescribing Tips for Patients with Renal Disease

- Nephrotoxic drugs should be avoided.
- Total number of drugs should be kept to a minimum.
- Ideally, use those agents that do not require renal metabolism to an active form or renal excretion either of the drug or its active metabolites.

Table 5.10: Stages of renal impairment

Stage	*Description of kidney function/failure*	*Estimated glomerular filtration rate in%*
1	Normal	>90
2	Mild	60–80
3	Moderate	30–50
4	Severe	15–20
5	Established severe	<10

- Close monitoring is required to check for any deterioration in renal function following the addition of new medicine.
- If there is no obvious alternative to a renally cleared drug, consider its therapeutic index. Drugs with a narrow therapeutic index should be avoided or should be used with all necessary precautions. Only drugs with a wide therapeutic index may be used with a reduced dose or frequency of administration. Therapeutic drug monitoring may be needed to guide dosing.
- Loading doses may be needed in renal impairment as the time to steady-state concentration is related to the half-life of the drug. The half-life is prolonged by reduced clearance, and so the time to steady state is longer. In this situation, the loading dose will help to achieve the desired effect on time.

While caution is essential, it is also important not to undertreat patients with renal impairment. Specialist help will be invaluable.

For patients on dialysis, new prescribers should not tackle these patients alone but should seek guidance by specialist medical colleagues.

Drugs in Renal Transplantation

Immunosuppressant therapy is needed in transplant patients to reduce the risk of rejection. Azathioprine, mycophenolate mofetil, calcineurin inhibitors (e.g. ciclosporin, tacrolimus) and basiliximab are commonly used drugs. Withholding or stopping these drugs can cause transplant rejection and therefore they should not be stopped without consultation with the medical team treating patient's other diseases.

Drugs requiring dose reduction in renal impairment

- Antidiabetic medicines
- Digoxin
- Aminoglycosides
- Opioids
- Amphotericin
- Teicoplanin
- Azathioprine
- Cotrimoxazole
- Morphine

Drugs contraindicated in severe renal failure

- NSAIDs
- Vancomycin
- Aminoglycosides
- Lithium
- Metformin
- Ethambutol
- Amphotericin B
- Glibenclamide
- Tetracycline

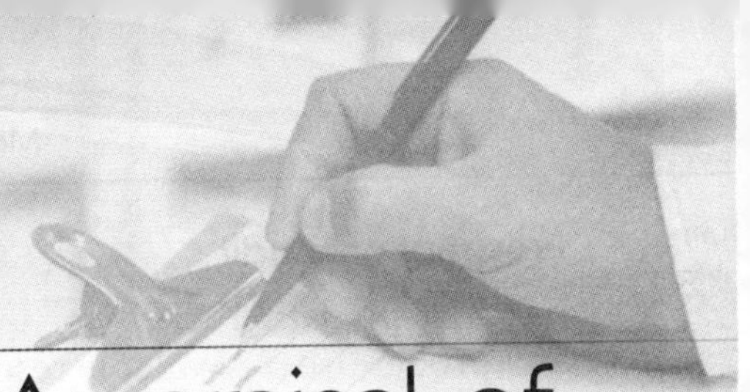

Chapter

6 Critical Appraisal of Prescription and Prescription Audit

Prescription is a written medico-legal document for therapeutic intervention by the treating physician reflecting his approach towards safe prescribing and providing quality health care to the patient.

Critical appraisal is a technique for systematic assessment and evaluation of the strength of factual claims, reliability and relevance of prescription which helps professionals to take an appropriate clinical decision, enhancement of skill and training of medical students.

Critical Appraisal Tool (CAT)

CAT is the structured checklist that allows assessment of the quality and completeness of a prescription against the standard criteria.

S. No.	*Parameters*	*Yes/No*
1.	Prescriber's Name, Professional degree, Address and Telephone number/e-mail address	
2.	Patient name, age, sex, weight and address.	
3.	Date of writing the prescription.	
4.	Diagnosis – provisional or definite/final.	
5.	Symbol Rx	
6.	Appropriate and relevant investigations needed for diagnosis and treatment	
7.	The drug name is written in clear and legible handwriting. In handwritten prescription, it should be in capital letters	
8.	Generic name of the drug is used (As per erstwhile MCI notification)	
9.	The drugs prescribed are correct as per the diagnosis	
10.	Type of drug preparation or formulation, dose, route of administration, frequency, duration of treatment and directions for use are written correctly	
11.	Is there overprescribing or underprescribing	
12.	Is there any contraindicated ingredient included in prescription	
13.	Is there irrational prescribing	
14.	Is there any abbreviation used	
15.	Are the instructions and advice for follow up to the patient given correctly and completely	
16.	Are the instructions to the pharmacist given and are complete	
17.	Is the role of non-pharmacological measure is given	
18.	Do's, Don'ts and referrals are mentioned (wherever required)	
19.	Prescriber's signature with date and registration number with a regulatory body	

Prescription Audit

It is a systematic review for quality improvement process with predefined criteria and proper use of available resources to deliver the right medicine to the right person in a health care system. Prescription auditing is also an educational activity that should be done regularly.

Objectives of Audit

1. To evaluate the effectiveness of a therapy
2. To prevent problems related to medication
3. To control drug cost
4. To update practitioners.

WHO's Definition of Rational uses of Drugs (RUD)

"Rational use of drugs requires that patients receive medications appropriate to their clinical needs, in doses that meet their own individual requirements for an adequate period of time, and the lowest cost to them and their community" (WHO, 1985). Irrational prescriptions are likely to increase the cost and duration of the treatment unnecessarily. The WHO has reported that around 50% of all medicines are inappropriately prescribed, dispensed, or sold. This is seen to have potential implications on health care budgets as almost 25–70% of worldwide health care expenditure is spent on medicines. Such inappropriate use of drugs also leads to the emergence of drug interactions, drug resistance, and adverse drug reactions. It ultimately increases the mortality, morbidity, and financial burden on the patients.

Core Drug use Indicators

WHO has standardized and evaluated a number of indicators which measures performance in three related areas and are grouped into three categories, namely:

a. Prescribing indicators
b. Patient care indicators
c. Health facility indicators

a. ***Prescribing indicators:*** The prescribing indicators measure the performance of health care providers in five key areas related to the appropriate use of medicines.
   1. *Average number of drugs per prescription*

Aim: To assess the extent of polypharmacy
Optimum value: <2
Mathematical expression: (p) = y/x
x = Total clinical encounters for which data was collected
y = The total number of medicines prescribed for the total encounters

Note: The combination medicines should be counted as one.

   2. *Percentage of drugs prescribed by generic name*

Aim: To measure prescriber's tendency to prescribe medicines using generic or international nonproprietary name (INN)

Optimum value: 100%
Mathematical expression: (g) = d/y × 100
d = The total number of medicines prescribed in the INN format
y = Total number of medicines prescribed

3. *Percentage of encounters with an antibiotic prescribed*

Aim: To assess the frequency of antibiotic prescribing among primary health care (PHC) providers
Optimum value: <30%
Mathematical expression: (b) = f/x × 100%
f = Number of prescriptions with antibiotic prescribed
x = Total number of encounters

Note: The WHO/ INRUD have provided a list of medicines which should usually be categorized into the group of antibiotics and have advised that where researchers deviate markedly from this categorization, this should be mentioned in the study's methodology. The WHO classification of antibiotics has been outlined in Table 6.1. The determination should be made whether dermatologic creams and eye care products should be regarded as antibiotics.

Table 6.1: World Health Organization antibiotic classification

Medicines usually classified as antibiotics	*Medicines which should usually not be classified as antibiotics*
Penicillins	Antifilarials
Anti-infective dermatological agents	Antischistosomals
Anti-infective ophthalmological agents	Antileprosy drugs
Antidiarrheal drugs with streptomycin, neomycin, nifuroxazide or combinations	Antituberculosis drugs
Other antibacterials	Antifungals
	Antiamoebic and antigiardiasis drugs
	Antileishmaniasis agents
	Antimalarials
	Antitrypanosomal drugs

4. *Percentag of injections per prescription*

Aim: To describes the frequency with which injectable forms of medicines are prescribed
Optimum value: <20%
Mathematical expression: (j) = t/x × 100%
t = Number of drug use encounters in which injection is prescribed
x = Total number of encounters

Note: Immunizations are not counted as injections

5. *Percentage of drugs prescribed from the essential drugs*

Aim: To access whether prescribing practices conform to drug use policy as pertaining to the use of essential medicines list (EML).
Optimum value: 100%.
Mathematical expression: (k) = m/y × 100%
m = Number of medicines prescribed from EDL
y = Total number of medicines prescribed

Note: The concept of EML use is built on the premise that the use of a limited number of well-known and cost-effective medicines can lead to better health care, uninterrupted long-term medicines supply and more easy and approachable access to products. In assessing this indicator, investigators must obtain a copy of the reference EML (national or facility-based) for comparison of prescribed medicines.

B. Patient-care Indicators

- Average consultation time
- Average dispensing time
- Percentage of drugs actually dispensed
- Percentage of drugs adequately labelled
- Patients' knowledge of correct dosage.

C. Health Facility Indicators

- Availability of copy of essential drug list in all OPDs
- Availability of key drugs.

Thus, periodic prescription audits may encourage the error-free prescribing and may ensure that drug therapy meets the current standard of care.

Chapter

7

Legal and Ethical Aspects of Prescribing Drugs

Who can Prescribe In India?

A registered medical practitioner (RMP) is the only authorized person to prescribe allopathic medicines that includes an allopathic doctor with minimum MBBS, a dentist with minimum BDS, and a veterinarian with minimum BVSc degree registered with the respective State Medical/Dental/Veterinary Council. To date persons with unrecognized degrees, nurse, pharmacist, or quacks are not authorized by the government of India to prescribe allopathic drugs. However, in some countries like the UK, USA, and Australia after specialized training, health personnel other than doctors are permitted to prescribe drugs to treat some conditions.

Ethical Principles of Care

Ethics is the system of moral principles that apply values and judgment to the practice of medicine. Ethical principles that guide the successful approach to treatment are autonomy, honesty, beneficence, justice, avoidance of conflict of interest and the pledge to do no harm. Ethics is an integral part of medical practice. The clinician has multiple roles to play like diagnosis, treatment and to give relief and comfort to the patients. "The right conduct of the physician towards patient's care is correct caring for the patient."

What is "Good Prescribing"?

Considering the fact that when many drugs are available to treat a particular disease, good prescribing includes maximum effectiveness, minimum risks, minimum costs with due respect to the patient's choice of therapy. Involve the patient in the decision making by giving him different options, e.g. modality of therapy for breast cancer or how far to proceed with the treatment of terminal illnesses. The patient should be informed about the potential adverse effects and cautions. The empathic clinician plays important role in helping patients and their families to bear the burden of serious illness and death.

What is Model Prescription Format?

A proper format for prescription writing ensures the appropriate use of drug and helps in minimizing errors. In order to avoid ambiguity, erstwhile MCI has issued a model prescription format in 2015 which a registered medical practitioner has to follow.

Doctor's Name:
Qualification (e.g. MBBS,MD)
Reg. no.:.................................... (ALLOPATHY)
Full Address, Contacts: (Telephone No. E-mail etc.)
Date:
Name of Patient ....
Address*..
Age and Sex...Weight** ....

R_x

1. Name of Medicine***
   Strength, dosage instruction, duration, and total quantity***
2. -do-
3. -do-

Doctor's Signature
Stamp

DISPENSED

Date ....Pharmacist......................

Name of Pharmacy ....

City ....

*Postal Address / E-mail /Mobile Number
** Pediatric Patients
*** In CAPITAL letters only

Minimum size of the Prescription blank should be (a) 14 × 21 cm (A5 size) and (b) XI × XI cm

In this format, in addition to all elements of ideal prescription as described in part 1, there is a place on the left bottom side of the prescription for entry by the dispenser after the doctor's signature and seal. Here chemist or pharmacist should write the quantity of drugs dispensed along with signature, date and name of the pharmacy/ medical store and city. This is especially important for the dispensing of drugs causing dependence.

Professional Misconduct of Prescribing

The prescription is considered as a legal record of drug administration; hence it must be a clear document providing factual evidence of what occurred, as well as accountability of the concerned parties. These parties would include not only the prescriber but also the professional who dispensed or administered the drug.

Professional misconduct of prescribing includes:

- Illegible handwriting or writing drugs details in small letters difficult to understand in the prescription.
- Not writing generic drugs
- Proper and effective communication with the patient about drugs prescribed is not taken care of.
- Prescribing drugs of one particular brand available at a particular pharmacy for commercialization.
- Accepting gifts from a pharmaceutical company to write their drugs.
- Writing drugs or supplying drugs to addicts.
- Violation of drug acts and regulations
- Running a shop to sell drugs
- Involvement in an advertisement of any drug for its promotion in print or social media.

If the doctor is found guilty of professional misconduct NMC may exert disciplinary action on the doctor or their name may be erased from medical register either temporarily or permanently. A doctor cannot practice if his/ her name is removed from the medical register.

Laws that Govern Prescriptions in India

Prescription is the heart of medical therapy: A legal document governed by the following laws:

- The Indian Medical Council Act, 1956
- The Indian Medical Council (Professional Conduct, Etiquette & Ethics) Regulations, 2002
- The Drugs and Cosmetics Act, 1940 and Rules 1945
- The Narcotic Drugs and Psychotropic Substances Act, 1985 and Rules 1987
- Drugs (Price Control) Order, 1995
- The Drugs and Magic Remedies (Objectionable Advertisements) Act, 1954 and Rules 1955

Chapter

8

E-Prescribing

E-Prescribing or electronic prescribing is the system of transmitting prescription and related information electronically by the prescriber to the patient and the dispenser on mobile phone or computer. An electronic prescription can be used in place of paper prescription to get medicines from the pharmacy. Concept of e-prescribing is gaining momentum in the present era and being widely adopted because of its recognition as one of the most promising tools to reduce medication errors due to paper prescriptions.

Benefits of E-prescribing

1. It is potentially convenient and advantageous in eliminating subjective errors due to illegible handwriting and incorrect medicine dispensing.
2. Electronic prescribing potentially ameliorates the adverse drug events and drug-drug interactions in the ambulatory care settings due to prescription check software which provides automated alerts and reminders at the time of prescribing.
3. E-prescribing systems automatically highlight patient allergies making prescribers aware of them.
4. Each prescription can be linked with a high-quality database to check that the drug prescribed is appropriate for a particular age, gender, comorbidity and laboratory investigation reports so that patient safety is ensured by reducing fatal mistakes.
5. E-prescribing systems prompt the prescriber to choose the most appropriate drug available and quickly add common instructions, leading to faster prescribing and dispensing correct doses.
6. Prescribers are enabled to receive a cost-effective recommendation of drugs and patients get financial benefits.
7. E-prescribing eliminates the risk of tampering or altering prescriptions.
8. Chances of incorrect interpretation of electronic orders by a pharmacist are very less.
9. Increased access to patient medication records, and improved pharmacy workflow.
10. Easy refilling of medicine from pharmacy by getting clinician's permission electronically particularly in cases of chronic diseases reduces the waiting time of the patients.
11. Mobile devices and wireless networks enable prescribers to modify or edit prescriptions from the places wherever they are.

12. Misinterpretation or omission of critical information is identified even before processing the prescription ensuring quality of care.
13. Reconcile medication history quickly across multiple settings of care and increased patient satisfaction.
14. Patient's medical record and office billing system, if integrated electronically can give information about treatment expenditure to the patient and hospital administrators.
15. The technology also benefits by bringing significant financial savings attributed to less office space, better efficiency with lesser staff and fewer claims and penalties due to a reduction in medicine errors.

Challenges of E-prescribing

1. The high initial cost to establish and implement an e-prescribing system.
2. Additional efforts are required to train all concerned members to adopt effective integration of this technology with the office management, scheduling system, billing systems, and electronic medical records for successful e-prescribing.
3. Protection of the security and confidentiality of medical records and personal identifiable information (PII) of the patient is of extreme importance.
4. Poor designing of e-prescribing software can cause unintended harm to the patients.

Though electronic prescribing is safe and efficient, it should not be considered as a substitute for personal attention to the individual patient by the health professional.

Chapter

9 Off Label Prescribing

Background

Prescription of a licensed medicine for a use that is not approved by a regulatory agency and not included in the drug label or in the product information is off label prescribing. The practice is common and legal in many countries. The regulatory bodies do not have the legal authority to regulate the practice of the medicine, and the physician may prescribe a drug off label for standard care to the patients.

Off label prescribing includes the use of an approved drug for the following unlabeled conditions:

- *Indication*, e.g. anticancer drug mitomycin is indicated for the treatment of gastric and pancreatic carcinoma also used for the treatment of lung, bladder, breast, cervical, and other carcinomas not approved by the US FDA.
- *Age group:* Lack of paediatric indications on drug labels often lead to off label prescribing, hence many drugs indicated for adults are also prescribed off label in the paediatric population.
- *Dose strength:* When a drug is approved at a dose of 500 mg but prescriber advises other than approved dose.
- *Route of administration*, e.g. drugs approved by IV route and given by intrathecal route e.g. pentazocine, gentamicin.
- *Dosage form:* When a medication is approved as a tablet or capsule and is used topically or when tablets are given as suspension to children.

Medicine Areas with Frequency of Off Label Prescribing

Due to the fact that certain populations like the elderly, children and pregnant women and certain health conditions like mental health disorders, malignancy and patients in intensive care units are not always included in clinical trials, off label prescribing is frequently seen based on the latest evidence. Furthermore in mental disorders in addition, the similarity of symptoms between disease states also contributes to off label prescribing.

Pros and Cons of Off Label Prescribing

Physicians practice medicine based on their professional judgment keeping in mind both the safety and efficacy of the medication not limited to official, approved indications. Many new therapies and evidence have emerged out of off label prescribing, however, for pharmaceutical companies to get approval for new uses of old drugs by clinical testing is time-consuming and costly. Some such off label uses are scientifically valid giving treatment benefits to patients. Paclitaxel initially approved for treating ovarian cancer, was found to be effective for treating breast cancer when used off label. After the publication of reports showing its effectiveness in breast cancer, it was later approved by regulatory bodies. Gabapentin an antiepileptic drug is used for bipolar disorder, fibromyalgia, headache, hot flashes, and restless leg syndrome as off label.

On the other hand, inappropriate use of off label drugs is a cause of concern when it is used without risk-benefit analysis. The safety with off label use has attracted much attention when caused serious adverse effects. For example "Fen-phen" an unapproved combination of fenfluramine and phentermine used for weight loss resulted in heart valve disease.

Though off label drug use is very common throughout the world, most often this is done without adequate scientific data. To date, there is no uniform regulatory framework available to help clinicians to assess the appropriateness of off label prescribing.

Proposed Points of Consideration for Appropriateness of Off Label Prescribing

Off label prescribing is not considered legal in India even when it does not violate ethical guidelines or other safety regulations. There is a need of universal guidelines to maximize the benefits and to minimize the harm from off label prescribing. We propose the following points:

- Make certain that it would better serve the patient's needs than a licensed alternative.
- Take patient's or their representative's consent for their treatment being done by the unlicensed drug. Explain the reasons why medicines are not licensed for their proposed use and make him/her understand this newer implication.
- Check clinical suitability and cost effectiveness of off label use of the drug. The decision must not be based on potentially biased information or commercial gain.
- Collect sufficient evidence to demonstrate the medication's safety and efficacy for that particular patient.
- Document the clinical management plan clearly in terms of which drug is chosen and the reason for choosing it, continuous monitoring of the treatment and progress of the treatment in detail.

Circumstances Motivating Off Label Prescribing

Physicians prescribe drugs off label for a variety of situations all aiming at better patient care:

1. Nonavailability of a suitable licensed medicine that will treat the patient's disease. For example, metformin in polycystic ovarian syndrome a hormonal disorder common in women of reproductive age.
2. In children when licensed medicine fails to treat a condition or symptom but a medicine licensed for the same condition or symptom in adults found effective.
3. The dosage specified for a licensed medicine when not found to correct the disease.

Table 9.1: Examples of some off label uses

Drug	*On label*	*Off label*
Propranolol	Hypertension, thyrotoxicosis	Anxiety
Amitriptyline	Depression	Neuropathic pain, prophylaxis migraine
Prazocin	Hypertension	Nightmares
Gabapentin	Epilepsy	Hot flushes, restless leg syndrome
Metformin	Diabetes mellitus	PCOD
Divalproex	Antiepileptic	SSRI-induced headache
Escitalopram	Depression	Bipolar disorder
Bupropion	Depression	Bipolar disorder
Sertalazine	Depression	Bipolar disorder
Venlafaxine	Depression	Bipolar disorder
Duloxetine	Depression	Anxiety
Trazodone	Depression	Sleep disturbances

4. The patient asks for a formulation of a drug that is not specified in an applicable license.
5. Due to a temporary shortage in supply of a suitable licensed medicine, other suitable approved drug which is not indicated for this condition is used to treat the patient.
6. The prescribing forms part of a properly approved research project.
7. In case of emergency when there is an urgent need for a new drug or indication, and there is a report of nonefficacy of labeled drug in certain demographics.
8. In cases when label drug is costly for the patient and physician prescribes another drug which is cost effective though not having a label for that particular use. For example, bevacizumab a low-priced drug approved for the treatment of metastatic colorectal cancer is used off label for age-related macular degeneration in place of approved drug ranibizumab which is very costly.

When Off Label use is Illegal or Problematic?

1. Violation of ethical guidelines or other safety regulations.
2. Nonavailability of adequate data regarding drug safety and effectiveness for the off label use.
3. Physician promoting off label uses through mass media such as the television and internet.
4. Drug's manufacturer promoting a drug for an indication which has not received marketing authorization from the government agency, even if significant scientific evidence exists for that unapproved indication.

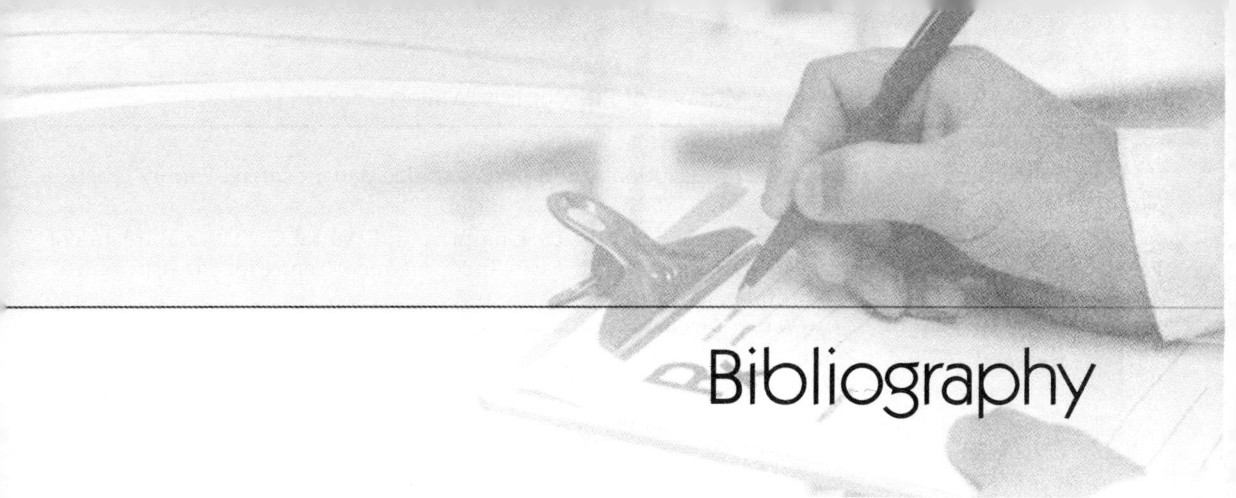

Bibliography

1. Ackermann E, Litt J and Morgan M. Prescribing Drugs of Dependence in General Practice, Part C1: Opioids (2017).
2. Aronson JK, Henderson G, Webb DJ and Rawlins MD. A Prescription for Better Prescribing (2006).
3. Bennet PN, Brown MJ, Sharma P. Clinical Pharmacology, 11th edn, 2012, Charchill Livingstone, Edinburg.
4. Buxton ILO. Principles of prescription order writing and patient compliance. Goodman and Gilman's The Pharmacological Basis of Therapeutics, 12th edn, 2011, McGraw-Hill, New York.
5. Cash JC and Glass CA (Eds.). Family Practice Guidelines, 2017, Springer Publishing Company.
6. De Vries TPG, Henning RH, Hogerzeil HV, Fresle DA, Policy M, and World Health Organization. (1994). Guide to Good Prescribing: a practical manual (No. WHO/DAP/94.11).
7. Guidelines of Programmatic Management of Drug Resistant Tuberculosis In India 2019 by Revised National Tuberculosis Control Programme, Central TB Division, Directorate General of Health Services, Ministry of Health and Family Welfare, Nirman Bhawan, New Delhi.
8. Hitchings A, Lonsdale D, Burrage D and Baker E. The top 100 drugs: Clinical Pharmacology and Practical Prescribing (2018). Elsevier Health Sciences.
9. Hogerzeil HV (editor), et al. Teacher's Guide To Good Prescribing (No. WHO/EDM/PAR/ 2001.2).
10. International Ethical Guidelines For Health Related Research Involving Humans by CIOMS in collaboration with WHO 2016.
11. Jameson LJ, Fauci A, Kasper D, Hauser S, Longo D & Loscalzo J. Harrison's Principles of Internal Medicine, 20 th edn, 2018 (Vol.1 & Vol.2), McGraw-Hill Education.
12. Katzung BG, Masteres SB, Trevor AJ (Eds): Basic and Clinical Pharmacology, 14th edn, 2018, New Delhi, McGraw-Hill, Education (India).
13. Kennan K, Mathiharan K (editors). A Textbook of Medical Jurisprudence and Toxicology, 25th edn, 2016 Lexis Nexis, Reed Elsevier, Gurgaon, Haryana, India.
14. National Formulary of India (NFI 2016). Indian Pharmacopoeia Commission, Ministry of Health and Family Welfare, Directorate General of Health Services, New Delhi, 2015.
15. National List of Essential Medicines (NLEM 2015) Govt of India, Ministry of Health and Family Welfare, Directorate General of Health Services, New Delhi, 2015.
16. Papadakis MA, McPhee SJ and Rabow MW. Current Medical Diagnosis and Treatment, 2020, Lange McGraw-Hill, New York.
17. Proposed guidelines for prescription writing and handling for drugs having misuse or abuse potential, proposed by FDA, Goa at the stakeholders meeting held on 23rd September, 2009.
18. Rang HP, Ritter JM, Flower RJ, Handerson G. Rang and Dale's Pharmacology, 8th edn, 2020, Elsevier, Churchill Livingstone Edinburgh.

19. Teichman PG and Caffee AE. Prescription writing to maximize patient safety. Family Practice Management, vol 9 no. (7), 2002.
20. VenkateshS, Chauhan LS, Gadpayle AK, Jain TS, Ghafur A and Wattal C. National treatment guidelines for antimicrobial use in infectious diseases. India: National Centre for Disease Control, MOHFW, Government of India, (2011). 1–64.
21. WHO. How to Investigate Drug Use in Health Facilities: Selected Drug Use Indicators: EDM Research Series No. 007. 1993. [Last accessed on 2015 May 05]. Available from: http://www.apps.who.int/medicinedocs/en/d/Js2289e/
22. Woodfield G, Phillips BL, Taylor V, Hawkins A and Stanton A. Essential Practical Prescribing. (2016). John Wiley & Sons.

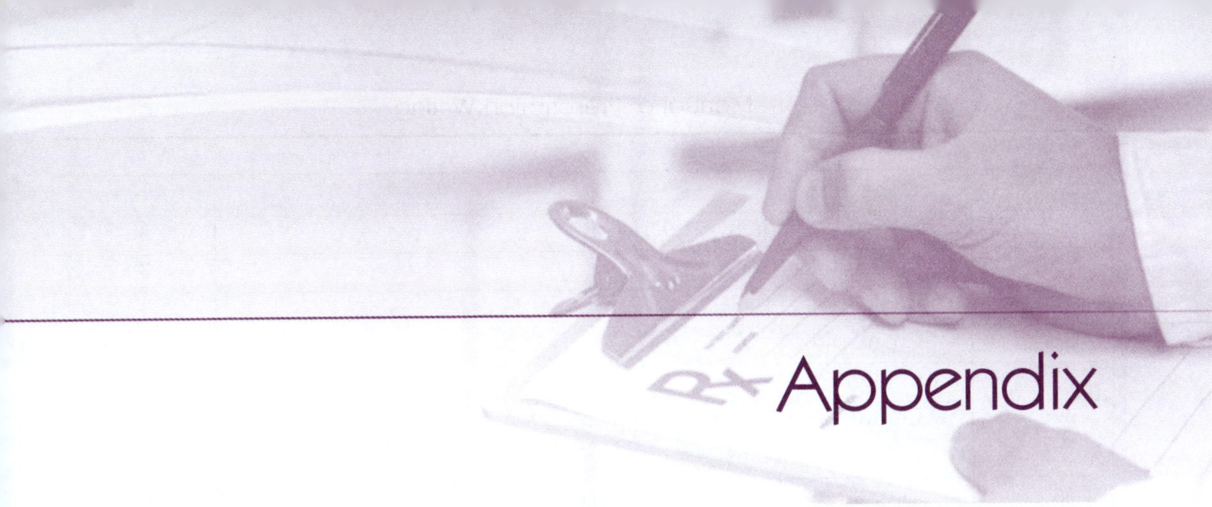

Appendix

Alphabetical List of Diseases

Contd.

Contd.

Contd.

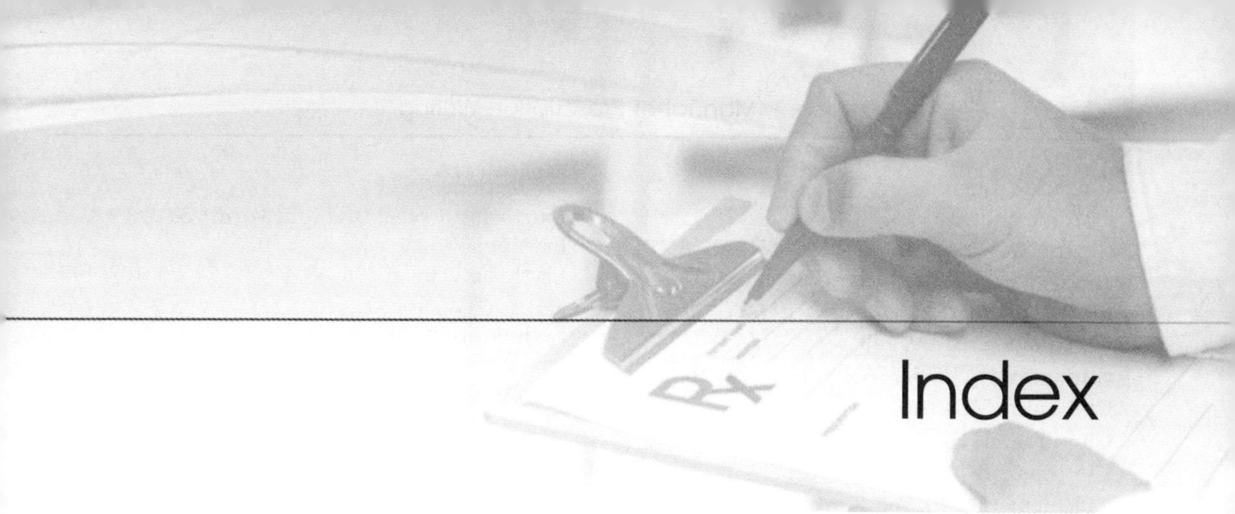

Index